AF870419

INDEPENDENT STUDY GUIDE

AHIMA CHDA 2026

Study Guide 2026

✓ Aligned to official exam objectives
✓ Adversarially verified practice questions
✓ Complete preparation resource

Meridian Certification Press
An imprint of Big Five Killer

AHIMA CHDA 2026
Study Guide 2026

Published by Meridian Certification Press
An imprint of Big Five Killer

ISBN 9798259502499 (Paperback)
ISBN 9798259502505 (Hardcover)

Copyright © 2026 Big Five Killer. All rights reserved.

This study guide is an independent publication and is not affiliated with, authorized by, endorsed by, or in any way officially connected with AHIMA (American Health Information Management Association). All certification names and trademarks are the property of their respective owners.

AI Disclosure. Portions of this book were drafted with the assistance of large language models. All content was reviewed, edited, and verified by the editorial team at Meridian Certification Press. Practice questions and answer explanations underwent adversarial accuracy review.

Accuracy Commitment. If you believe you have found an error, please report it to meridian@bigfivekiller.online.

First edition, May 2026.

Contents

How to Use This Guide

This study guide is built around the AHIMA Certified Health Data Analyst (CHDA) exam blueprint for the 2026 testing cycle. The CHDA credential validates a candidate's ability to acquire, manage, analyze, interpret, and report data that drives healthcare decision-making across clinical, operational, financial, and regulatory contexts. Earning it requires more than memorization. The exam tests judgment: which data source to trust, which method to apply, how to communicate results to a non-technical executive, and when a finding is clinically actionable versus statistically interesting but operationally trivial.

The guide is organized into seven chapters that map to the major CHDA domains: data governance and stewardship, data architecture and management, data quality, healthcare analytics and statistical methods, reporting and visualization, regulatory compliance, and clinical classification systems. Each chapter opens with the estimated exam weight, follows with explicit learning objectives, and presents a body of substantive material drawn from authoritative sources — the HIPAA Privacy and Security Rules, the 21st Century Cures Act information-blocking regulations, the Office of the National Coordinator's interoperability standards, the National Center for Health Statistics' ICD-10-CM Official Guidelines, the Centers for Medicare and Medicaid Services' Inpatient Prospective Payment System rules, and AHIMA's own data quality management model. Every chapter ends with two to three exam tips, three to five key concepts, and five review questions with annotated answers.

A 50-question practice exam follows the chapters. It is calibrated to mirror the proportion of questions you should expect from each domain on the live exam. Treat the practice exam as a diagnostic, not a final dress rehearsal. After taking it, score yourself by domain, not just overall. A 70 percent overall score with a 40 percent score on data governance is a warning that needs targeted remediation before exam day.

A four-week and an eight-week study plan are provided in Appendix C. Choose based on your work schedule and your baseline familiarity with the material. If you already work as a clinical data analyst, the four-week plan is realistic. If you are transitioning from coding, billing, or general HIM, plan on eight weeks and budget extra time for the analytics and statistics chapter.

On exam day, you have four hours to complete 150 multiple-choice questions, of which 130 are scored and 20 are unscored pretest items. You will not be told which is which. Pace yourself at roughly 90 seconds per question. Flag questions you are uncertain about and return to them; do not let a single hard item consume five minutes. The exam is delivered through Pearson VUE, online-proctored or at a physical test center. Bring two forms of identification, arrive thirty minutes early, and confirm your testing environment meets Pearson's requirements at least 48 hours before your appointment.

A passing score is scaled — AHIMA does not publish the raw passing percentage because difficulty varies across forms — but candidates who consistently score 75 percent or higher on the practice exam in this guide have a strong likelihood of passing on the first attempt. If you score below 65 percent on the practice exam, consider deferring your appointment by two to four weeks.

Data Governance and Stewardship

Exam weight: approximately 15 percent

0.1 Learning Objectives

After completing this chapter, you will be able to:

- Distinguish between data governance, data stewardship, and data management, and identify the organizational roles responsible for each.
- Apply the AHIMA Information Governance Adoption Model (IGAM) framework to evaluate an organization's governance maturity.
- Develop and enforce data definitions, business glossaries, and metadata standards.
- Identify the legal, regulatory, and ethical obligations that constrain how healthcare data may be used, shared, and retained.
- Recognize when a data request requires escalation to a data governance committee or to compliance.

0.2 Content

Data governance in healthcare is the formal exercise of authority and control over the management of data assets. It is not the same as data management, which refers to the operational handling of data — extraction, transformation, loading, and storage. Governance sets policy; management executes it. A useful working definition, derived from the Data Management Association International (DAMA) Body of Knowledge and adapted by AHIMA for the healthcare context, is that data governance establishes who can take what action, upon what data, in what situations, using what methods.

The CHDA exam expects candidates to know that data governance in a healthcare provider organization is typically structured around three layers. At the top sits a Data Governance Council, often chaired by a Chief Data Officer, Chief Medical Information Officer, or Chief Health Information Officer, with members drawn from clinical leadership, finance, compliance, legal, information technology, and health information management. The council sets policy, approves data definitions, resolves cross-functional disputes about data ownership, and authorizes major data initiatives such as enterprise data warehouse builds or vendor contracts that involve protected health information.

The middle layer consists of Data Stewards. A data steward is the operational owner of a defined data domain — for example, the patient demographics steward, the lab results steward, or the financial transactions steward. Stewards are accountable for the definitions, quality, and appropriate use of their domain. They are usually subject-matter experts embedded in the relevant business unit, not centralized data team members. The CHDA exam frequently tests the distinction: data stewards do not necessarily own the technical systems that store the data, but they own the meaning, the quality criteria, and the use authorization.

The bottom layer is the Data Custodian. Custodians are typically IT personnel responsible for the physical and logical security of the data — the database administrators, the cloud platform engineers, the backup operators. They execute the access controls that governance and stewardship have defined.

AHIMA publishes the Information Governance Adoption Model (IGAM), which provides a maturity assessment across ten competencies including strategic alignment, accountability, awareness and adherence, information lifecycle management, and information integrity. The model uses a five-level maturity scale ranging from Level 1 (minimal or no formal governance) through Level 5 (transformational, where information governance is embedded in strategic decision-making). The CHDA exam may present a scenario describing an organization's practices and ask you to identify the corresponding IGAM maturity level. As a rule, the presence of a written policy moves an organization from Level 1 to Level 2. The presence of documented enforcement mechanisms moves it to Level 3. Documented measurement of compliance against the policy moves it to Level 4. Active use of the measurements to drive continuous improvement is Level 5.

A core artifact of data governance is the enterprise data dictionary, sometimes called the business glossary. This is the authoritative record of every defined data element used in reporting, analytics, or operations. A good entry includes the element name, a precise business definition, the system of record, the data type and allowed values, the steward, the date the definition was last reviewed, and any synonyms or aliases. The exam tests the principle that two different reports producing two different numbers for the same metric — for example, "average length of stay" — is almost always a definitional problem, not a data quality problem. Length of stay can be calculated as discharge date minus admission date, or as the count of midnights spent in the facility, or by excluding observation hours, or by excluding leave-of-absence days. Until the organization commits to one definition and enforces it through the data dictionary, every report will tell a different story.

Healthcare data governance must also address the legal and regulatory frame. The Health Insurance Portability and Accountability Act (HIPAA) of 1996, codified at 45 CFR Parts 160 and 164, establishes the federal floor for the privacy and security of protected health information. State laws may impose additional restrictions, particularly around mental health records, substance use disorder records (governed federally by 42 CFR Part 2), and HIV-related information. A governance program must inventory the applicable laws for each jurisdiction in which the organization operates and translate them into operational policies on access, disclosure, retention, and breach response.

The 21st Century Cures Act, signed in 2016, and the implementing regulations issued by the Office of the National Coordinator for Health Information Technology (ONC) in 2020 — the Cures Act Final Rule — introduced the concept of information blocking. As of the rule's effective date, healthcare providers, health information networks, and certified health information technology developers are prohibited from engaging in practices that are likely to interfere with the access, exchange, or use of electronic health information, except as required by law or covered by one of eight defined exceptions: preventing harm, privacy, security, infeasibility, health IT performance, content and manner, fees, and licensing. The CHDA candidate must understand that an analytics request to share patient-level data with an outside care partner is no longer governed only by HIPAA but also by the Cures Act information-blocking framework. A reflexive refusal that would once have been considered prudent privacy practice may now constitute information blocking.

Data stewardship in practice involves continuous activity: reviewing data quality dashboards, adjudicating data quality incidents, approving access requests that exceed standing role-based permissions, and updating definitions when business needs change. A common exam scenario describes a clinician requesting access to an entire patient population's data for a quality improvement project. The CHDA-correct response identifies the minimum necessary standard (45 CFR 164.502(b)) and requires the steward to evaluate whether de-identified data, a limited data set under a data use agreement, or a fully identified release with IRB or privacy board waiver is appropriate.

A mature governance program also addresses data lifecycle management. Every data element should have a defined retention period and a defined disposition method. Federal Medicare conditions of participation require retention of medical records for at least five years; state laws often require longer (typically seven to ten years; some states require retention until the patient reaches a defined age plus a number of years for pediatric records). Financial records have their own retention requirements under tax law. Quality reporting submissions must be retained for at least six years under the False Claims Act statute of limitations. The governance program must reconcile these requirements and document a unified retention schedule. Destruction of records before the end of the retention period — even by accident — can create regulatory and litigation exposure.

Finally, governance addresses ethical considerations that extend beyond legal compliance. The use of predictive models in clinical decision-making raises questions about algorithmic bias, particularly when models are trained on historical data that reflects disparities in care. A governance program should require model validation across demographic subgroups, ongoing monitoring of model performance, and transparency to clinicians about how a model arrives at a recommendation. The Office of the National Coordinator's Health Data, Technology, and Interoperability: Certification Program Updates, Algorithm Transparency, and Information Sharing rule, finalized in late 2023 and effective in stages through 2025, imposes specific transparency requirements on certified decision support interventions. The CHDA exam may test whether a candidate recognizes when an analytics deliverable crosses from descriptive reporting into clinical decision support, triggering these additional obligations.

> **Exam Tip**
>
> When a question describes a conflict over a metric definition, the correct answer almost always involves the data dictionary or the data steward, not a technical fix in the warehouse.

Exam Tip

Information blocking under the Cures Act applies to healthcare providers, not only to vendors. A refusal to share data with a competing health system, when the patient has authorized the exchange, can trigger penalties under 42 USC 300jj-52.

Exam Tip

Records retention is governed by the longest applicable requirement. If state law requires seven years and federal Medicare conditions require five, retain for seven.

Key Concept

Data governance sets policy; data stewardship enforces it in a specific domain; data custody secures the underlying systems. The three roles are distinct and rarely held by the same person.

Key Concept

The Information Governance Adoption Model (IGAM) progresses from policy existence (Level 2) to policy measurement (Level 4) to continuous improvement (Level 5). A written policy without measurement is not mature governance.

Key Concept

The minimum necessary standard at 45 CFR 164.502(b) is the operational test for every analytics access decision involving PHI. De-identified data is preferred when it answers the question.

Key Concept

A limited data set, defined at 45 CFR 164.514(e), permits use of certain identifiers (dates, geographic information larger than a street address) but requires a Data Use Agreement.

Key Concept

The Cures Act Final Rule changed the default from "share only when explicitly required" to "share unless explicitly excepted." Eight defined exceptions exist; any other refusal risks an information-blocking finding.

0.3 Chapter Review Questions

Q1. A clinical research team requests dataset access containing patient names, dates of birth, and full street addresses for a population health study. The data governance council asks whether HIPAA permits the disclosure. Which response is correct?

A) The data can be shared as a limited data set if a Data Use Agreement is executed.
B) The data may be shared only under an authorization or an IRB-approved waiver, because full street addresses and names are direct identifiers.
C) The data can be shared without restriction because the request is for research.
D) The data can be shared as de-identified data if the dates of birth are removed.

Answer: B — A limited data set under 45 CFR 164.514(e) excludes direct identifiers including names and street addresses; what remains is dates and geographic information larger than a street address. For a research disclosure that includes names and full addresses, the covered entity needs a patient authorization or an IRB or privacy board waiver under 45 CFR 164.512(i).

Q2. Two operational reports show different "average length of stay" values for the same month. Investigation reveals one report uses calendar days (discharge date minus admission date) while the other counts midnights. Which corrective action should the CHDA recommend first?

A) Reprogram one of the reports to match the other.

B) Bring the discrepancy to the data steward and update the enterprise data dictionary with a single approved definition.
C) Escalate to the IT department as a data integration error.
D) Investigate whether one of the source systems is calculating dates incorrectly.

Answer: B — The discrepancy is a definitional, not a technical, problem. CHDA expects candidates to recognize that the data steward for the encounter domain owns the metric definition, and the resolution must be documented in the data dictionary before any report is reprogrammed; otherwise the same problem will recur with the next new report.

Q3. An organization has a written policy on data access controls, an enforcement mechanism through technical role-based controls, and conducts an annual audit comparing actual access logs against policy. The audit results are reported but no follow-up actions are taken. Which IGAM maturity level best describes this state?
A) Level 2 (developing)
B) Level 3 (defined)
C) Level 4 (managed)
D) Level 5 (transformational)

Answer: C — Level 4 corresponds to documented measurement of policy adherence. Movement to Level 5 requires active use of the measurement results to drive continuous improvement. Reporting without follow-up is the textbook indicator of Level 4 rather than Level 5.

Q4. Under the Cures Act information-blocking rule, a hospital refuses to send a patient's records to a competing health system that has been treating the patient for cardiology follow-up, citing concerns about commercial competition. Which statement is correct?
A) The refusal is permitted because the receiving entity is a competitor.
B) The refusal is permitted only if the patient has not authorized the disclosure.
C) The refusal is likely information blocking because competitive concerns are not among the defined exceptions.
D) The refusal is permitted under the security exception.

Answer: C — The Cures Act Final Rule defines eight exceptions to information blocking (preventing harm, privacy, security, infeasibility, health IT performance, content and manner, fees, licensing). Commercial or competitive considerations are not among them. Refusing exchange on competitive grounds, when the patient is the subject and treatment continuity is at stake, is the paradigmatic information-blocking violation.

Q5. A data steward and a data custodian disagree about whether to grant a new analytics platform read access to the patient demographics table. Who has authority to make the final decision under a standard healthcare governance structure?
A) The data custodian, because they manage the technical access controls.
B) The data steward, because they own the data domain's authorized use.
C) The IT director, because the request involves a technical platform.
D) The privacy officer, because PHI is involved.

Answer: B — The data steward owns the data domain and is accountable for authorizing use. The custodian implements the authorization technically but does not decide whether the use is appropriate. The privacy officer is consulted when HIPAA permissibility is uncertain, but routine access decisions for an internal analytics platform sit with the steward.

Data Architecture, Management, and Integration

Exam weight: approximately 18 percent

0.4 Learning Objectives

After completing this chapter, you will be able to:

- Distinguish between operational systems, data warehouses, data marts, data lakes, and lakehouse architectures, and identify the analytical use cases each is best suited to.
- Apply dimensional modeling principles (Kimball) and normalized modeling principles (Inmon) appropriately for healthcare reporting.
- Explain the structure and use of common healthcare data standards: HL7 v2, FHIR R4 and R5, CCDA, X12, and the USCDI.
- Design or evaluate an ETL or ELT pipeline that integrates clinical, administrative, and financial source systems.
- Manage master data, including the patient master index and the provider master file.

0.5 Content

Healthcare data architecture is shaped by two recurring tensions: the need for transactional systems optimized for speed and consistency at the point of care, and the need for analytical systems optimized for cross-encounter, cross-patient, and longitudinal query performance. The same database design cannot serve both well. The CHDA exam expects candidates to navigate this division comfortably and to know when a question is asking about the transactional side, the analytical side, or the integration layer between them.

Operational systems — the electronic health record, the laboratory information system, the radiology information system, the pharmacy management system, the patient accounting system, the human resources system — are typically built on row-oriented relational databases optimized for online transaction processing. Their schemas are normalized to third normal form or beyond. They handle thousands of small, fast transactions per second: a clinician orders a medication, a lab posts a result, a charge is captured. Querying them for analytical purposes is technically possible but operationally undesirable. Long-running analytical queries can slow transactional performance and degrade the user experience at the bedside. They also produce inconsistent results when run across changing data.

The data warehouse is the canonical answer to this problem. Bill Inmon, often called the father of the data warehouse, defined it as a "subject-oriented, integrated, time-variant, and non-volatile collection of data in support of management's decision-making process." The four properties matter. Subject-oriented means organized around business subjects (patient, encounter, claim) rather than around source applications. Integrated means harmonized: the same patient identifier across all source systems, the same code for "female" across all source systems, the same definition of "admission" across all source systems. Time-variant means every record carries time stamps that allow point-in-time reconstruction. Non-volatile means records are appended, not updated in place, so historical reports can be reproduced exactly.

Inmon's modeling approach is top-down: build a comprehensive, normalized enterprise data warehouse first, then derive dependent data marts for specific business areas. Ralph Kimball's competing approach is bottom-up: build dimensional data marts directly, organized around business processes, and let the union of marts form the enterprise warehouse through conformed dimensions. Kimball's star schema, with a central fact table surrounded by dimension tables, has become the dominant pattern for healthcare analytics because it is simple to query, performs well on aggregations, and maps naturally to the business questions clinicians and administrators actually ask.

A fact table in a healthcare star schema typically corresponds to a measurable event: an inpatient encounter, an outpatient visit, a medication administration, a lab result, a charge. Each row records the event's measurements (length of stay in days, total charges, lab result value) and foreign keys to the dimension tables that describe the context (which patient, which provider, which date, which diagnosis, which procedure). Dimension tables are denormalized for query performance. A patient dimension might have dozens of attributes (date of birth, sex, race, ethnicity, ZIP code, primary care provider, primary insurance) all in a single wide row.

Slowly changing dimensions are a particular challenge in healthcare. A patient's address, insurance, primary care provider, and even legal name can change over time. The CHDA exam expects familiarity with the three principal techniques. Type 1 overwrites the old value with the new value; this is appropriate for corrections of erroneous data but loses history. Type 2 preserves history by adding a new row with an effective date range and a current-record flag; this is the standard approach for healthcare attributes that change for legitimate reasons. Type 3 adds a new column to hold the previous value; this is appropriate when only one prior value matters and the change is rare.

A data mart is a subject-area subset of an enterprise data warehouse, often optimized for a specific user community: a finance mart for revenue cycle analytics, a quality mart for clinical performance measures, a population health mart for risk stratification. Marts can be physical (separate databases) or virtual (views over the warehouse). The advantage of dedicated marts is performance tuning and simplified semantics for the user community; the disadvantage is the risk of definitional drift away from the enterprise warehouse if governance is weak.

The data lake emerged in the mid-2010s as an alternative pattern, particularly attractive when the volume, variety, and velocity of data outpaces the schema-on-write discipline of a warehouse. A lake stores data in its raw form, often in cloud object storage (Amazon S3, Azure Data Lake Storage, Google Cloud Storage) as Parquet, ORC, or Avro files. Schema is applied on read rather than on write. The advantage is flexibility: any data can be ingested without prior modeling. The disadvantage is the well-documented risk of a "data swamp" — a lake without governance becomes unusable because no one knows what is in it or whether it is trustworthy.

The lakehouse architecture, popularized by Databricks with the Delta Lake format and by other vendors with Apache Iceberg and Apache Hudi, attempts to combine the flexibility of the lake with the reliability and governance of the warehouse. Lakehouses support ACID transactions on data lake files, schema enforcement and evolution, and time travel queries. For CHDA purposes, the candidate should know the names, the general capabilities, and the fact that the lakehouse is currently the architecture of choice for new builds at most large health systems and payers.

Integration patterns connect the operational and analytical layers. Extract, Transform, Load (ETL) is the classical pattern: data is pulled from source systems, transformed in a staging area, and loaded into the warehouse. Extract, Load, Transform (ELT) reverses the order: raw data is loaded first and transformed within the destination platform, exploiting modern data platforms' computational power. ELT has become more common as cloud data warehouses (Snowflake, BigQuery, Databricks SQL, Redshift) have made in-database transformation cheap and fast.

Healthcare adds an integration layer above generic ETL: standards-based interfaces. HL7 v2 has been the dominant clinical messaging standard since the early 1990s, and is still pervasive for ADT (admission, discharge, transfer), ORM (order), ORU (result), and other transaction-level messages. It is a pipe-and-hat-delimited text format that is verbose, idiosyncratic, and lacks formal semantics, but it is universally supported. Any CHDA candidate has seen something like `MSH|^~\&|SENDING_APP|...` in a log file and recognized it as an HL7 v2 message header.

The HL7 Consolidated Clinical Document Architecture (C-CDA) was developed to support exchange of structured clinical documents in XML. It is the format underlying the Continuity of Care Document and the Transition of Care Document required for meaningful use and now Promoting Interoperability. CCDA is verbose, complex, and uses the SNOMED CT, LOINC, RxNorm, and ICD-10-CM code systems to bind clinical concepts to standardized terminologies.

FHIR (Fast Healthcare Interoperability Resources) is HL7's current standard, designed for the modern web. FHIR R4 was published in 2019 and is the version required by the Cures Act and by CMS for the Patient Access API. FHIR R5 was published in 2023. The standard organizes clinical data into "resources" — Patient, Encounter, Observation, Condition, Procedure, MedicationRequest, and approximately 150 others — each addressable by a URL and serializable in JSON or XML. FHIR's RESTful API model has made it the practical foundation for patient-facing apps, third-party developer ecosystems, and increasingly for backend integration.

The United States Core Data for Interoperability (USCDI) is the ONC's specification of the minimum data classes and elements that certified health IT must support. USCDI version 1 was finalized in 2020; subsequent versions have expanded the scope. Version 3 added social determinants of health elements (e.g., food insecurity, housing instability). Version 4 added pediatric vital signs and substance use elements. The CHDA exam may test whether a candidate can identify whether a given data element is or is not in the current USCDI, which has direct implications for whether the data is available through standard FHIR APIs.

For administrative and financial data, HIPAA mandates the use of X12 EDI transaction standards. The 837 transaction conveys claims; 835 conveys remittance advice; 270/271 are eligibility inquiry and response; 276/277 are claim status; 278 is referral and authorization. The CHDA exam may present a scenario involving claims data and expect the candidate to recognize the source transaction and its structure.

Master data management addresses entities that appear across multiple systems and must be unambiguously identifiable. The Patient Master Index (sometimes Enterprise Master Patient Index, EMPI) is the most critical: every system uses its own internal patient identifier, but enterprise analytics requires a single identity per patient regardless of source. EMPI software uses probabilistic and deterministic matching across attributes (name, date of birth, sex, social security number, address) to link source identifiers to a single enterprise identifier. Duplicate records and overlay errors are the two principal failure modes: a duplicate is one person represented by two enterprise identifiers; an overlay is two people erroneously merged into one identifier. The latter is much more dangerous because it can result in one patient's clinical history being applied to another patient at the point of care.

The Provider Master File serves the analogous purpose for clinicians and is increasingly important as quality reporting moves to clinician-level attribution. The National Provider Identifier (NPI), a ten-digit number issued by CMS, is the federally mandated identifier and the foundation of any provider master.

> **Exam Tip**
>
> When a scenario asks whether a real-time clinical use case should be served from the operational system or the warehouse, the answer is almost always the operational system. The warehouse is non-volatile and updated in batch; it cannot reflect the patient's current state.

> **Exam Tip**
>
> Slowly changing dimension Type 2 is the default for healthcare patient attributes. Type 1 is reserved for correction of errors, not legitimate change of state.

> **Exam Tip**
>
> FHIR R4 is the version required by federal regulation as of 2026. R5 is published but not yet mandated. If a question asks which version is "required," answer R4 unless the question specifies a future state.

> **Key Concept**
>
> Inmon builds an enterprise normalized warehouse first; Kimball builds dimensional marts first and integrates through conformed dimensions. Most modern healthcare implementations are Kimball-style at the user-facing layer.

> **Key Concept**
>
> A patient overlay (two patients merged into one record) is more dangerous than a duplicate (one patient in two records). EMPI quality programs prioritize overlay prevention.

> **Key Concept**
>
> USCDI defines the minimum data set certified health IT must support via FHIR APIs. The version number matters because new elements (e.g., social determinants of health in USCDI v3) become available only as the version advances.

> **Key Concept**
>
> ETL transforms before loading; ELT loads then transforms. Cloud data platforms have made ELT the default for modern healthcare data builds.

> **Key Concept**
> HL7 v2 is still pervasive for transaction-level messaging (ADT, ORM, ORU); FHIR is the standard for document-level and API-based exchange.

0.6 Chapter Review Questions

Q1. A health system is designing a new analytic platform and needs to retain the historical insurance plan associated with each encounter, even though a patient's current insurance may change. Which slowly changing dimension technique is most appropriate for the patient dimension's insurance attribute?

A) Type 0 (no change tracked)
B) Type 1 (overwrite)
C) Type 2 (new row with effective date range)
D) Type 3 (previous-value column)

Answer: C — Type 2 preserves the full history of insurance assignments by inserting a new row each time the value changes, with effective_start and effective_end dates and a current_flag. This allows encounter-level joins to reflect the insurance in force at the time of service, which is required for accurate financial reporting.

Q2. Which standard is required by the ONC Cures Act Final Rule for certified electronic health records to support patient and population services APIs?

A) HL7 v2.5.1
B) C-CDA R2.1 only
C) FHIR R4
D) X12 837

Answer: C — The Cures Act Final Rule requires certified health IT to support standardized APIs based on FHIR Release 4, including the Bulk Data Access (Flat FHIR) capability for population-level access. C-CDA is required for document exchange but not for the API requirement.

Q3. An EMPI audit identifies two records in the enterprise data warehouse with the enterprise ID 1004727. The two records have different dates of birth and different sexes, but were merged based on a matching name and a matching old address. Which classification applies?

A) Duplicate record
B) Overlay error
C) Acceptable probabilistic match
D) Data quality outlier

Answer: B — An overlay error occurs when two distinct patients are erroneously merged into a single enterprise identity. This is the more dangerous EMPI failure mode because clinical data from one patient may be applied to another at the point of care. Differing dates of birth and sexes are red flags that the match should never have occurred.

Q4. A claims analyst needs to know what services were performed for a member during a specified date range. Which X12 transaction is the source data for this analysis?

A) 270 (eligibility inquiry)
B) 837 (claim)
C) 835 (remittance advice)
D) 278 (referral)

Answer: B — The 837 transaction conveys claims, including service line detail with procedure codes, diagnosis codes, dates of service, and billed amounts. The 835 conveys the payer's response, which is useful for reimbursement analysis but does not by itself report the services provided.

Q5. Which architectural choice would best support a use case requiring point-in-time reconstruction of a patient's record as of a specific historical date?

A) The operational EHR with a real-time query
B) A non-volatile, time-variant data warehouse
C) A virtual data mart over the operational EHR
D) A snapshot file produced manually each month

Answer: B — Inmon's definition of a data warehouse includes non-volatility (records are not updated in place) and time-variance (every record carries time stamps). Together these properties enable accurate point-in-time reconstruction. The operational EHR overwrites historical state for many fields; manual snapshots are limited to the dates snapshots happened to be taken.

Data Quality Assessment and Improvement

Exam weight: approximately 15 percent

0.7 Learning Objectives

After completing this chapter, you will be able to:

- Apply the AHIMA Data Quality Management Model and its ten characteristics of data quality.
- Design and execute data quality assessments using profiling, sampling, and rule-based validation.
- Identify the root causes of common healthcare data quality defects in registration, coding, charge capture, and clinical documentation.
- Construct data quality dashboards and remediation plans.
- Distinguish between intrinsic and extrinsic data quality dimensions and prioritize improvements appropriately.

0.8 Content

Data quality is not a property of data in the abstract; it is a property of data with respect to a defined use. The same dataset may be high-quality for one purpose and unfit for another. A registration database that records a patient's stated address at the moment of arrival is high-quality for billing — the bill goes to the address the patient gave — but may be low-quality for population health work that needs the patient's current residential address.

The AHIMA Data Quality Management Model, originally published in 1998 and revised most recently to align with current information governance work, identifies ten characteristics of data quality. The CHDA exam tests recognition of these characteristics, often by presenting a scenario in which one characteristic is violated and asking the candidate to name it.

The ten characteristics are: accuracy (the data correctly represents the real-world fact); accessibility (authorized users can obtain the data when they need it); comprehensiveness (all required data elements are present); consistency (the same data element has the same value when reported by different systems); currency (the data is up to date); definition (the data element has a clear, agreed-upon meaning); granularity (the level of detail is appropriate to the use); precision (the data captures the necessary level of exactness); relevancy (the data answers the question being asked); and timeliness (the data is available within the time frame required).

These characteristics can be grouped into intrinsic quality (accuracy, consistency, definition, granularity, precision) and extrinsic or contextual quality (accessibility, comprehensiveness, currency, relevancy, timeliness). Intrinsic quality is about the data itself; extrinsic quality is about the fit between the data and the use case. An exam scenario describing a report that is "always at least three days behind" is a timeliness defect. A scenario describing two fields that "should match but never do" is a consistency defect.

Data profiling is the systematic examination of a dataset to characterize its content, structure, and quality. A profile of a column typically reports the percentage of nulls, the count of distinct values, the minimum and maximum, the mean and median for numeric data, the most frequent values, the data type distribution if the column is loosely typed, and the conformance to expected patterns (e.g., a date column where some values do not parse as dates). Profiling tools such as Great Expectations, dbt tests, Soda, Talend Data Quality, Informatica Data Quality, and Microsoft Purview have become standard. The CHDA candidate should know the general capability rather than tool-specific commands.

Rule-based validation supplements profiling by encoding business rules that the data must satisfy. A few examples that appear in healthcare quality programs: every encounter must have a discharge disposition; admission date must precede discharge date; for live discharges, length of stay must be at least one day; mortality flags must be consistent with discharge dispositions of "expired" or "donor"; sex-specific diagnoses must be consistent with patient sex; pediatric diagnoses must be consistent with patient age. Each rule produces a count of violations, and the violation count over time produces a quality trend.

Healthcare data quality defects cluster in a small number of upstream sources. Registration is the largest single source of demographic and insurance defects. The registration encounter is brief, the registrar is under throughput pressure, the patient may not have or know all the required information, and the consequences of a defect (delayed bill, payer rejection, identity error) are often invisible to the registrar. Improving registration quality requires both technology (real-time eligibility checks, address verification services, identity proofing tools) and process (defined rework procedures, supervisor review of high-risk fields, feedback from downstream consequences back to the registrar).

Coding is the principal source of diagnosis and procedure data quality defects. Coding accuracy depends on clinical documentation: the coder can only code what the physician documents. Clinical documentation improvement (CDI) programs employ specialists who review records concurrently, identify ambiguous or incomplete documentation, and query the physician for clarification. The CDI query process is governed by AHIMA and ACDIS guidelines and is heavily tested on the CHDA. Compliant queries must be non-leading, present multiple reasonable options when offering choices, and be retained as part of the medical record. The leading query is the most common compliance defect: a query like "Was the patient's pneumonia due to gram-negative bacteria?" leads the physician toward a single answer and inflates the case mix improperly. The compliant alternative offers a range of plausible options including "unable to determine."

Charge capture is the principal source of revenue cycle data quality defects. Missed charges, duplicate charges, charges to the wrong account, and charges that fail edit checks all produce financial loss or rework. A 2 percent missed charge rate on a $500 million net patient revenue base represents $10 million of leakage. Data quality programs in revenue cycle typically focus on charge reconciliation: comparing the orders and services documented in the EHR against the charges posted to the patient accounting system, identifying gaps, and investigating root causes.

Clinical documentation quality is broader than CDI's coding focus. A clinical note must be timely, legible (a residual concern even in the electronic record because of templated text and copy-forward errors), accurate, and complete. Copy-and-paste use, sometimes called "note bloat," is a particular concern: a clinician may bring forward an old assessment that is no longer accurate, creating a note that misrepresents the patient's current status. The Joint Commission has published standards (record-of-care chapter) addressing documentation expectations, and the Office of Inspector General has investigated copy-forward billing fraud where outdated documentation is used to justify higher-level evaluation and management codes.

A data quality dashboard makes quality measurable and visible. For each defined quality dimension, the dashboard reports a current rate, a trend, a target, and a status indicator. Examples: percent of encounters with a discharge disposition (target: 100 percent; current: 99.4 percent; trend: improving); percent of inpatient cases with a principal diagnosis code (target: 100 percent; current: 99.9 percent; trend: stable); percent of registrations with a verified address (target: 95 percent; current: 87 percent; trend: declining; status: red). The dashboard is operational only if it drives action. AHIMA's model calls for a defined remediation cycle: identify the defect, perform root cause analysis, design a corrective action, implement, measure the effect, and either sustain or iterate.

Sampling is necessary when full-population analysis is infeasible. A 200-record random sample of a year's inpatient encounters can support a coding audit with reasonable confidence intervals. Stratified sampling, in which the population is partitioned by a relevant variable (DRG family, payer, service line) and samples are drawn from each stratum, is appropriate when the rates of defects are believed to vary by stratum. Convenience sampling — auditing the records that happen to be easy to access — is not appropriate because it produces biased estimates.

A particular point of emphasis for the CHDA: data quality is a continuous program, not a project. A one-time scrub of the patient master may improve quality temporarily, but without continuous monitoring and continuous improvement of the upstream processes that introduce defects, the rates will drift back to the original baseline within months. The exam frequently presents a scenario in which an organization runs a one-time cleanup project and then claims success; the CHDA-correct answer identifies the need for ongoing monitoring and process improvement.

> **Exam Tip**
>
> When a scenario describes a data quality problem, identify which of the ten characteristics is at issue before proposing a fix. The exam often tests recognition of the specific characteristic.

> **Exam Tip**
>
> Leading queries are the most common CDI compliance defect on the exam. A query that names a single diagnosis or that presents only one clinical option is non-compliant.

> **Exam Tip**
>
> A copy-forward note that includes outdated assessment statements is a documentation quality defect with both clinical and compliance dimensions. The exam treats this as a documentation integrity issue.

> **Key Concept**
>
> Data quality is defined with respect to use. The same data can be fit for billing and unfit for population health, or vice versa.

> **Key Concept**
>
> The ten characteristics of the AHIMA Data Quality Management Model are: accuracy, accessibility, comprehensiveness, consistency, currency, definition, granularity, precision, relevancy, and timeliness.

> **Key Concept**
>
> Compliant CDI queries are non-leading, offer multiple reasonable options, and are retained as part of the medical record per AHIMA and ACDIS guidelines.

> **Key Concept**
>
> Sustainable data quality requires upstream process improvement, not just downstream cleanup. A one-time scrub without process change will regress.

0.9 Chapter Review Questions

Q1. A coder receives the following physician query: "The patient was admitted with elevated WBC and a positive blood culture. Was the patient septic?" Which characterization is correct?

A) The query is compliant because it cites clinical evidence.
B) The query is non-compliant because it is leading.
C) The query is non-compliant because it does not name a specific organism.
D) The query is compliant because it asks a yes-or-no question.

Answer: B — A compliant CDI query offers multiple reasonable options drawn from the clinical evidence and avoids suggesting a single answer. This query is leading because it presents sepsis as the only diagnostic possibility despite the presence of multiple plausible explanations (e.g., contaminant, localized infection without sepsis). A compliant version would offer sepsis, contaminant, localized infection, and "unable to determine" as options.

Q2. An analyst observes that a report of patients who appointment-no-showed is missing approximately 5 percent of expected records because the source system has a flag that is sometimes left blank. Which data quality characteristic is most directly violated?

A) Accuracy
B) Comprehensiveness
C) Granularity
D) Precision

Answer: B — Comprehensiveness addresses whether all required data elements are present. A missing flag value, when the flag is required for the report's purpose, is a comprehensiveness defect. Accuracy would describe a flag that is present but incorrect; precision would describe insufficient detail in a numeric measurement.

Q3. Which sampling strategy is most appropriate for a coding audit when DRG accuracy is believed to vary by service line?

A) Simple random sample of all encounters
B) Stratified random sample by service line
C) Convenience sample of records currently in the coder queue
D) Census of all encounters

Answer: B — Stratified random sampling improves precision when the parameter of interest varies by stratum. By drawing a sample from each service line, the audit can produce service-line-specific accuracy estimates rather than a single average that obscures variation. A simple random sample is less efficient because high-volume service lines dominate; a census is generally infeasible.

Q4. A data quality dashboard reports that 87 percent of registrations have a verified address. Management celebrates a 4-point improvement over last quarter. Which CHDA-aligned follow-up is most important?

A) Increase the target to 95 percent for next quarter.
B) Identify the registrars and registration sites driving the unverified 13 percent and conduct root cause analysis.
C) Reprogram the dashboard to exclude self-pay patients.
D) Issue a memo recognizing the improvement.

Answer: B — Sustainable improvement requires upstream process change. Identifying where the unverified registrations originate is the root-cause-analysis step that turns the dashboard from a scorecard into an operational improvement tool. Recognition is appropriate but secondary; raising the target without addressing the cause will not achieve it.

Q5. Two systems both report a count of "total admissions" for the previous month, but the numbers differ by 3 percent. Investigation shows one system counts observation patients who were converted to inpatient status as admissions on the date of conversion, while the other counts them as admissions on the original observation date. Which data quality characteristic is most directly at issue?

A) Definition
B) Accuracy
C) Timeliness
D) Granularity

Answer: A — Both systems are accurate against their own logic; they simply use different definitions of admission date. Definition is the characteristic that requires a clear, agreed-upon meaning for each data element. Resolution is through the data steward updating the enterprise data dictionary, not by changing either system unilaterally.

Healthcare Analytics and Statistical Methods

Exam weight: approximately 22 percent

0.10 Learning Objectives

After completing this chapter, you will be able to:

- Apply descriptive, diagnostic, predictive, and prescriptive analytics frameworks to healthcare problems.
- Select and apply appropriate measures of central tendency, dispersion, and association for healthcare data.
- Interpret common statistical tests including t-tests, chi-square, ANOVA, linear regression, and logistic regression.
- Calculate and interpret healthcare-specific rates and ratios: mortality rate, readmission rate, occupancy rate, case mix index, observed-to-expected ratios.
- Recognize the strengths and limitations of common predictive models used in risk stratification and quality measurement.
- Distinguish between statistical significance and clinical or operational significance.

0.11 Content

Healthcare analytics is the most heavily weighted domain on the CHDA exam, and for good reason. The credential exists to certify that the holder can do real analytical work on real healthcare data, not merely manage data infrastructure. The chapter is dense; budget time for it.

A common framing organizes analytics into four ascending types. Descriptive analytics asks what happened: counts, rates, averages, trends. Diagnostic analytics asks why it happened: drill-downs, segmentation, root-cause exploration. Predictive analytics asks what is likely to happen: regression, classification, time series forecasting. Prescriptive analytics asks what should be done: optimization, simulation, decision-support recommendations. The CHDA exam expects candidates to recognize each type when described and to know that most operational reporting is descriptive, most quality improvement work is diagnostic, most population health risk stratification is predictive, and most resource allocation recommendations are prescriptive.

Measures of central tendency describe the typical value of a distribution. The mean (arithmetic average) is the most familiar and is appropriate when the distribution is approximately symmetric and free of extreme outliers. The median (the middle value when sorted) is more robust to outliers and is preferred for skewed distributions. Length of stay is the classic healthcare example: a small number of very long stays pulls the mean upward, but the median represents the typical patient experience more accurately. The mode (the most frequent value) is rarely useful for continuous measures but is the appropriate central tendency for nominal categorical data — the mode of the principal diagnosis distribution is the most common reason for admission.

Measures of dispersion describe variability around the central tendency. The range is the difference between maximum and minimum and is highly sensitive to outliers. The interquartile range (IQR), from the 25th to the 75th percentile, is robust and pairs naturally with the median. The standard deviation is the square root of the variance and pairs naturally with the mean. For approximately normal distributions, about 68 percent of observations lie within one standard deviation of the mean and about 95 percent within two. Coefficient of variation (standard deviation divided by mean, expressed as a percentage) allows comparison of variability across measures with different units or scales.

Healthcare-specific rates and ratios appear repeatedly on the exam. The gross mortality rate is the number of inpatient deaths divided by the number of discharges (deaths plus live discharges) in a defined period, expressed as a percentage. The net mortality rate excludes deaths occurring within 48 hours of admission, on the grounds that those deaths are not attributable to the hospital's care; this distinction has become less emphasized in modern quality reporting but remains a CHDA exam topic. The cesarean section rate is cesarean deliveries divided by total deliveries. The infection rate for a defined infection (e.g., surgical site infection for a defined procedure) is infections divided by procedures, often multiplied by 1,000 or 100,000 to produce a more readable rate.

Readmission rate calculation requires care. The CMS Hospital Readmissions Reduction Program defines a readmission as an unplanned admission to an acute care hospital within 30 days of discharge from an index admission for one of six tracked conditions: acute myocardial infarction, COPD, heart failure, pneumonia, coronary artery bypass graft surgery, and elective primary total hip or knee arthroplasty. Each condition has a separate, risk-adjusted rate. The denominator is index admissions; the numerator is readmissions within 30 days. Planned readmissions (for example, planned surgical follow-up) are excluded by an algorithm based on procedure and diagnosis combinations. Risk adjustment accounts for patient-level factors (age, comorbidities, social risk factors as of FY 2024) so that hospitals serving sicker or more disadvantaged populations are not unfairly penalized.

Occupancy rate is the average daily census divided by the bed complement, expressed as a percentage. Inpatient service days are the patient-days actually provided. The average daily census is total inpatient service days divided by the number of days in the period. The bed complement is the total beds available (definition varies; sometimes licensed, sometimes set up and staffed). A 350-bed hospital with 290 inpatient service days per average day has an occupancy rate of 83 percent.

Case Mix Index (CMI) is the average DRG weight across a hospital's Medicare inpatient population (or a defined subset). CMI greater than 1.0 indicates a patient mix more resource-intensive than the national average; less than 1.0 indicates less resource-intensive. CMI is a critical financial metric because Medicare reimbursement is proportional to CMI times the hospital's base rate. CMI is also a critical analytic tool because changes in CMI over time can reflect changes in patient acuity, in case mix (which patients the hospital is admitting), or in documentation and coding practices. Separating these three drivers is a common CDI analytic exercise.

Observed-to-Expected (O/E) ratios are the workhorse of risk-adjusted quality reporting. The observed value is the actual count or rate in the population being evaluated. The expected value is the rate predicted by a risk-adjustment model applied to the same population. An O/E ratio of 1.0 indicates performance at the model's expectation. A ratio below 1.0 indicates better-than-expected performance (fewer adverse events than predicted). A ratio above 1.0 indicates worse-than-expected performance. Confidence intervals around the O/E ratio determine whether the difference from 1.0 is statistically significant. The CHDA exam tests interpretation: an O/E ratio of 0.85 with a 95 percent confidence interval of 0.78 to 0.93 indicates statistically significant better-than-expected performance because the interval excludes 1.0.

Statistical tests appear on the exam in scenario form, not as computational exercises. The Student's t-test compares means between two groups when the dependent variable is approximately normally distributed; the independent samples t-test compares two independent groups, the paired t-test compares matched observations (e.g., pre- and post-intervention measurements on the same patients). Analysis of variance (ANOVA) extends the t-test to three or more groups. The chi-square test of independence compares categorical distributions across two or more groups; a typical use is comparing readmission rates across payer categories. The Mann-Whitney U test (also called the Wilcoxon rank-sum) is the non-parametric counterpart to the t-test, used when the distribution is too skewed for parametric methods.

Linear regression models a continuous outcome as a linear function of one or more predictors. The coefficient on each predictor represents the average change in the outcome associated with a one-unit increase in the predictor, holding other predictors constant. R-squared reports the proportion of variance in the outcome explained by the model. Healthcare uses include modeling length of stay as a function of patient and clinical factors, modeling total cost as a function of DRG and risk score.

Logistic regression models a binary outcome as a function of predictors. The coefficient on each predictor, exponentiated, is the odds ratio: the multiplicative change in the odds of the outcome associated with a one-unit increase in the predictor. An odds ratio of 1.5 indicates that the odds increase by 50 percent per unit of predictor. Logistic regression is the most common method for healthcare risk stratification and is the basis for most CMS risk-adjusted quality measures. Model discrimination is typically evaluated using the c-statistic (also called the area under the receiver operating characteristic curve, AUC). A c-statistic of 0.5 is no better than chance; 0.7 is acceptable; 0.8 is good; 0.9 is excellent. Most CMS risk-adjustment models achieve c-statistics in the 0.65 to 0.75 range, reflecting the inherent difficulty of predicting acute clinical events.

Model calibration is the alignment between predicted and observed probabilities. A well-discriminating model can still be poorly calibrated if it systematically overpredicts or underpredicts. Calibration is evaluated using a calibration plot or the Hosmer-Lemeshow goodness-of-fit test, which compares observed and expected outcomes within deciles of predicted risk. Calibration is critical for clinical decision support because clinicians act on absolute risk, not relative risk.

The distinction between statistical and clinical significance is essential. A study with a very large sample may detect a 0.1 percent difference in mortality between two treatments as statistically significant (p less than 0.05), but a 0.1 percent difference may not be clinically meaningful. Conversely, a clinically important effect may fail to reach statistical significance in a small study. The CHDA candidate is expected to interpret findings in both dimensions: report the magnitude of the effect, the precision (confidence interval), and the clinical or operational meaning, not just the p-value.

Predictive models in healthcare are increasingly used for risk stratification: identifying patients at high risk of readmission, mortality, deterioration, or high cost so that interventions can be targeted. The Elixhauser and Charlson comorbidity indices remain widely used administrative-data risk adjusters. The LACE index (Length of stay, Acuity of admission, Comorbidity, Emergency visits in the past six months) predicts readmission. The HCC (Hierarchical Condition Categories) model is the Medicare Advantage risk adjustment model and the basis for shared savings calculations in many value-based contracts. Newer machine learning models (gradient-boosted trees, neural networks) often achieve higher discrimination than logistic regression but at the cost of interpretability and, sometimes, calibration.

Fairness in predictive models is a current and growing concern. A model that performs well on average can perform poorly for specific demographic subgroups, and historical data may encode disparities that the model perpetuates. Best practice and emerging regulation expect model validation across race, ethnicity, sex, age, payer, and language subgroups, with documented action when subgroup performance falls below an acceptable threshold. The ONC's 2023 transparency rule for predictive decision support interventions imposes documentation requirements; the FDA's framework for AI/ML-based software as a medical device imposes additional requirements when the model is regulated as a device.

> **Exam Tip**
>
> When length of stay or cost data appear in a scenario, the median is usually the better measure of central tendency because the distribution is right-skewed.

> **Exam Tip**
>
> An O/E ratio's statistical significance is determined by whether the confidence interval excludes 1.0. A ratio of 0.9 with an interval of 0.85 to 1.05 is not statistically significantly better than expected.

> **Exam Tip**
>
> Discrimination (c-statistic) and calibration are distinct properties of a predictive model. The exam tests recognition that a well-discriminating model can still be miscalibrated.

> **Key Concept**
>
> The four-tier analytics framework (descriptive, diagnostic, predictive, prescriptive) is the standard CHDA classification. Most healthcare operational reporting sits in the descriptive and diagnostic tiers.

> **Key Concept**
>
> CMS readmission measures are 30-day, all-cause, unplanned admissions following index admissions for six tracked conditions, risk-adjusted for patient characteristics.

> **Key Concept**
>
> Logistic regression with c-statistic between 0.65 and 0.75 is typical for healthcare risk-adjustment models. Higher c-statistics in vendor marketing materials warrant skepticism unless the model is validated on independent data.

> **Key Concept**
> Case Mix Index is the average DRG weight; changes can reflect patient acuity, case mix, or documentation/coding, and separating these is a standard analytic task.

> **Key Concept**
> Statistical significance is necessary but not sufficient for action. Effect magnitude and clinical or operational meaning must be reported alongside p-values.

0.12 Chapter Review Questions

Q1. A hospital has 350 beds. In the month of June (30 days), the hospital recorded 9,135 inpatient service days. What is the occupancy rate, rounded to the nearest whole percent?
A) 26 percent
B) 75 percent
C) 87 percent
D) 95 percent

Answer: C — Average daily census equals 9,135 divided by 30, or 304.5. Occupancy rate equals 304.5 divided by 350, or 0.870, rounded to 87 percent. Memorize the formula: occupancy rate = (inpatient service days / days in period) / bed complement.

Q2. A risk-adjusted mortality model produces an observed-to-expected ratio of 0.82 with a 95 percent confidence interval of 0.71 to 0.94 for a hospital's annual cardiac surgery cases. Which interpretation is correct?
A) The hospital's performance is not statistically distinguishable from expected.
B) The hospital's performance is statistically significantly worse than expected.
C) The hospital's performance is statistically significantly better than expected.
D) The hospital's performance is exactly at expected.

Answer: C — An O/E ratio less than 1.0 indicates better-than-expected performance. The confidence interval of 0.71 to 0.94 excludes 1.0, so the difference is statistically significant. The CHDA exam expects candidates to interpret confidence intervals as a significance test in observational reporting.

Q3. A 2-by-2 comparison of readmission rates between two payer groups produces a chi-square statistic with p-value 0.03. The absolute difference in readmission rates is 0.4 percentage points. Which characterization is most aligned with CHDA reporting principles?
A) The difference is statistically significant and therefore meaningful for operational action.
B) The difference is statistically significant but its clinical or operational meaningfulness depends on the magnitude.
C) The difference is not statistically significant because the absolute difference is small.
D) The result is uninterpretable without the chi-square value.

Answer: B — Statistical significance and operational meaningfulness are distinct. A 0.4 percentage point difference, while statistically detectable in a large sample, may or may not justify operational action depending on the baseline rate, the cost of intervention, and the population size. CHDA reporting separates statistical from operational significance.

Q4. Which scenario is best matched to logistic regression as the analytic method?
A) Modeling length of stay as a function of patient characteristics.
B) Comparing average cost between two service lines.
C) Predicting the probability that a heart failure patient will be readmitted within 30 days.
D) Forecasting next month's total inpatient admissions from a time series of monthly admissions.

Answer: C — Logistic regression is the canonical method for modeling a binary outcome (readmitted or not) as a function of predictors. Length of stay is continuous and is modeled by linear regression. The cost comparison is a t-test scenario. The forecasting problem is best handled by a time-series method such as ARIMA or exponential smoothing.

Q5. A hospital's Case Mix Index has increased from 1.65 to 1.78 over twelve months. Which of the following is NOT a plausible explanation that the CHDA analyst should investigate?
A) The hospital is admitting more complex patients.

B) Clinical documentation has improved, capturing comorbidities that were previously underdocumented.
C) The proportion of low-acuity admissions has increased.
D) The CDI program has been expanded.

Answer: C — A CMI increase from 1.65 to 1.78 indicates a more resource-intensive case mix on average. A higher proportion of low-acuity admissions would push CMI downward, not upward, and is therefore not a plausible explanation for the observed increase. The other three are all plausible drivers and the standard CDI-versus-acuity decomposition is one of the most important analyses on this exam.

Data Reporting, Visualization, and Communication

Exam weight: approximately 13 percent

0.13 Learning Objectives

After completing this chapter, you will be able to:

- Design dashboards and reports that match user needs at the executive, operational, and analytic levels.
- Apply principles of data visualization to choose appropriate chart types and avoid misleading presentations.
- Communicate analytic findings effectively to clinical, administrative, and lay audiences.
- Distinguish between operational, tactical, and strategic reporting cadences.
- Manage report inventories and retire redundant or stale reports.

0.14 Content

A common failure mode of analytic teams is producing technically correct outputs that do not change any decision. The CHDA exam tests whether the candidate understands that reporting is a communication discipline, not just a data discipline. The output is the answer to a question, presented to a decision-maker, in time and form suitable to action.

Effective reporting begins with the audience and the decision. An executive viewing a Monday morning dashboard needs to know within thirty seconds whether anything requires attention this week. An operational manager needs to see today's queue, today's targets, and today's exceptions. A clinical service line director preparing a quarterly review needs trends, comparisons, and drill-downs. Each audience has different time pressures, different domain literacy, and different responses available. The same data may need to be packaged three ways.

Edward Tufte's principles, while now over forty years old, remain the dominant framework taught for visualization design and are tested on the CHDA. The principles include: show the data (maximize data-ink ratio, minimize non-data ink); avoid chartjunk (decorative elements that distract from the data); choose graphical forms appropriate to the data type; and respect graphical integrity (do not distort the data through visual exaggeration).

Chart type selection is rule-based for the common cases. Trends over time use line charts. Comparisons across categories use horizontal or vertical bar charts. Composition of a whole uses stacked bars (preferred) or pie charts (limited to a small number of slices with large differences). Distributions use histograms or box plots. Relationships between two continuous variables use scatter plots. Three-dimensional charts, exploded pie charts, and most spider or radar charts are best avoided in formal reporting because they impair quantitative judgment.

Common visualization errors that the CHDA exam may test include: truncated y-axis scales that exaggerate small differences; dual-axis charts that imply spurious correlations; pie charts with too many slices; misleading area encodings (a bar's height is the encoded value, not its area); and inconsistent color schemes across related charts. Color choices matter: red-green color schemes are inaccessible to viewers with the most common form of color blindness; heat maps should use color scales that vary in luminance, not only in hue.

Dashboard design follows additional principles. The most important indicator goes in the top-left (Western reading order). Indicators are grouped by topic. Status (red/yellow/green) is the fastest read but must be defined by explicit thresholds. Trend indicators (arrows or sparklines) communicate direction at a glance. Drill-down should be available but not required for the primary read. The CHDA candidate should be able to identify when a dashboard violates these principles: an executive dashboard that requires navigating three menus to find the headline number, or a dashboard whose colors mean different things on different pages, is poorly designed.

Operational, tactical, and strategic reporting differ in cadence and audience. Operational reports are produced daily, hourly, or in real time, and are consumed by frontline staff and managers; they support immediate decisions about staffing, workload, and quality. Tactical reports are produced weekly or monthly, and are consumed by managers and directors; they support resource allocation, performance management, and short-cycle improvement. Strategic reports are produced quarterly or annually, and are consumed by executive leadership and the board; they support long-cycle decisions about service line strategy, capital investment, and organizational direction.

A common pathology is the use of strategic-cadence content (quarterly trends, comparative benchmarks, multi-year forecasts) on an operational dashboard. Frontline staff cannot act on quarterly information; the content distracts from the operational signal. The reverse pathology — operational detail on an executive dashboard — is equally common. The CHDA candidate is expected to recognize the mismatch.

Effective communication of analytic findings follows a standard structure regardless of the medium: the bottom-line finding first; the evidence that supports it; the caveats and limitations; the recommended action; the next step required from the audience. For a written report, this maps to an executive summary, body, methods, and recommendations. For an oral briefing, it maps to a thirty-second opener, a five-minute body, and a clear ask. For a dashboard, it maps to the headline indicator, the supporting detail, the metadata footer with definitions and source, and the link to action.

A recurring CHDA exam theme is responsible reporting. Even technically correct analytics can mislead if presented without context. A 50 percent month-over-month increase in a rate is alarming until the absolute numbers are revealed to be two cases versus three. A statistically significant result with a p-value of 0.04 and a tiny effect size may not justify the operational change being proposed. The reporter has an obligation to provide the context that protects the audience from drawing the wrong conclusion.

Reports should not proliferate without governance. A report inventory tracks every active report by name, owner, audience, refresh cadence, last-accessed date, and underlying data sources. Reports not accessed in 90 days are candidates for retirement; redundant reports (multiple reports answering essentially the same question) are candidates for consolidation. Without inventory management, analytic teams accumulate dozens or hundreds of reports, each of which represents an ongoing maintenance cost and a definitional risk.

Report distribution must respect access controls. A report containing PHI must be delivered only to recipients authorized to view that PHI. Email distribution of clear-text PHI reports has been a recurring source of HIPAA breaches; secure portal distribution with role-based access is the recommended pattern. Even aggregate reports may be subject to small-cell suppression rules if the cells represent identifiable populations. CMS's de-identification guidance generally suppresses cells with fewer than 11 patients in claims data analyses, though specific thresholds vary by program.

Self-service reporting tools (Tableau, Power BI, Qlik, Looker, modern BI platforms) have shifted some report production from analytic teams to business users. This shift has both benefits and risks. The benefit is faster turnaround for routine questions and reduced backlog on the analytic team. The risk is definitional drift: business users may produce reports that diverge from enterprise definitions, undermining consistency. The CHDA-aligned response to this risk is governance: a certified dataset layer with enforced definitions, a clear separation between certified and exploratory content, and ongoing literacy training for self-service users.

> **Exam Tip**
>
> When a question describes a dashboard that requires multiple clicks to find the headline number, the design defect is the violation of the principle that the most important indicator should be immediately visible.

> **Exam Tip**
>
> A pie chart with more than five or six slices is almost always wrong. A bar chart is the safer choice for comparison across many categories.

> **Exam Tip**
>
> Cell suppression for small populations (typically n less than 11) is a standard de-identification practice in CMS public reporting and a common exam topic.

> **Key Concept**

> Reporting cadence must match audience action: operational, tactical, or strategic. Mismatches degrade both the report and the decision.

> **Key Concept**
> A dashboard's most important indicator goes in the top-left position by Western reading-order convention. Status colors must be defined by explicit thresholds.

> **Key Concept**
> Self-service reporting requires a certified semantic layer to prevent definitional drift away from enterprise standards.

> **Key Concept**
> Effective analytic communication leads with the bottom-line finding, follows with the evidence, caveats, and recommended action, and closes with the next step required.

0.15 Chapter Review Questions

Q1. An executive dashboard shows monthly readmission rates over twelve months as a line chart with the y-axis ranging from 14.5 percent to 16.0 percent. A reader concludes that readmissions are highly volatile. What design choice most directly contributes to this misinterpretation?
A) The chart should be a bar chart, not a line chart.
B) The truncated y-axis exaggerates small differences.
C) The time period is too long.
D) The chart lacks a title.

Answer: B — A y-axis that does not begin at zero, when used with a tightly scaled range, visually exaggerates the magnitude of variation. Tufte's graphical integrity principle calls for axis scales that do not distort the data. The standard practice for rate charts is either a zero-based scale or a clearly labeled break.

Q2. A public reporting program publishes facility-level outcomes for an oncology procedure. Cells with fewer than 11 patients are suppressed. What is the principal reason for this rule?
A) Statistical instability of small-sample rates.
B) Risk of re-identifying individual patients.
C) Compliance with the HIPAA Security Rule.
D) Reduction of report production cost.

Answer: B — Small-cell suppression is principally a re-identification protection. With small numbers, the combination of a facility, a condition, and other public attributes can narrow the population to a single identifiable patient. Statistical instability is a real concern but is typically addressed through confidence intervals or asterisks, not suppression.

Q3. A nurse manager wants a dashboard showing today's patient flow: arrivals, discharges pending, beds available. Which reporting cadence is appropriate?
A) Operational (real-time or near-real-time)
B) Tactical (weekly)
C) Strategic (quarterly)
D) Ad hoc (on request)

Answer: A — Patient flow management requires immediate signal; the decisions (assigning beds, expediting discharges, calling in additional staff) happen on the same shift. Operational dashboards are designed for this cadence. Tactical and strategic content would be of no use for the manager's immediate decisions.

Q4. A self-service reporting environment has been deployed and within six months has accumulated 1,400 distinct reports created by business users. Many appear to answer similar questions with slightly different definitions. Which governance response is most consistent with CHDA principles?
A) Disable self-service and require all reports to come through the analytic team.

B) Establish a certified dataset layer with enforced definitions and maintain a report inventory with retirement criteria.
C) Allow all reports to remain because business users own their work.
D) Move all reports into a single shared folder.

Answer: B — Self-service is valuable but requires governance to prevent definitional drift. A certified semantic layer ensures that any user-built report rolls up to enterprise-consistent definitions. A report inventory with retirement criteria controls proliferation. Disabling self-service is a regression that pushes the bottleneck back to the analytic team.

Q5. Which chart type is most appropriate for showing the distribution of inpatient length of stay across all discharges in a quarter?

A) Pie chart by primary payer.
B) Line chart over time.
C) Histogram or box plot.
D) Scatter plot of length of stay against admission date.

Answer: C — Histograms and box plots are designed to display the distribution of a continuous variable. A pie chart by payer answers a different question (composition by category). A line chart over time displays a trend, not a distribution. A scatter plot would display a relationship rather than a distribution.

Regulatory Compliance, Privacy, and Security

Exam weight: approximately 10 percent

0.16 Learning Objectives

After completing this chapter, you will be able to:

- Apply the HIPAA Privacy Rule, Security Rule, and Breach Notification Rule to analytic data uses.
- Distinguish between de-identified data, limited data sets, and protected health information.
- Implement appropriate access controls, audit logs, and minimum-necessary practices.
- Recognize the obligations of the HITECH Act, the Cures Act, 42 CFR Part 2, and state-level privacy laws.
- Manage research data uses under the Common Rule and HIPAA research provisions.

0.17 Content

The HIPAA Privacy Rule, codified at 45 CFR Part 164 Subpart E, governs the use and disclosure of protected health information (PHI) by covered entities (health plans, healthcare clearinghouses, and most healthcare providers) and their business associates. The CHDA exam tests operational application of the rule, not its full legal text. The candidate should be able to identify when a use or disclosure is permitted, when it requires authorization, and when it triggers minimum-necessary analysis.

Permitted uses without authorization include treatment, payment, and healthcare operations (TPO). Treatment is the provision of care to a patient. Payment is the activities undertaken to obtain reimbursement. Healthcare operations is a defined list of activities including quality assessment and improvement, case management, fraud and abuse detection, and general administrative activities. Most internal analytics on operational data falls within healthcare operations. The CHDA candidate is expected to recognize that running a readmission analysis to drive a quality improvement project is healthcare operations, not research, and therefore does not require authorization or IRB review.

Research is the systematic investigation designed to develop or contribute to generalizable knowledge. The legal distinction between research and quality improvement is the intent to generalize. A quality improvement project to reduce readmissions at one's own hospital is operations; a study to publish findings about readmission reduction interventions in a peer-reviewed journal is research. The same activity can shift between categories based on the intent, and the CHDA exam tests recognition of the line.

Research uses of PHI require either (a) patient authorization, (b) an IRB or privacy board waiver of authorization under 45 CFR 164.512(i), (c) a limited data set with a Data Use Agreement, or (d) preparatory-to-research review (a representation by the researcher that the use is preparatory and that no PHI will be removed). The CHDA candidate should know that the IRB waiver requires the research to involve no more than minimal risk to privacy, that the research could not practicably be conducted without the waiver, that the research could not practicably be conducted without access to the PHI, and that adequate plans for protection and destruction are in place.

De-identified data, defined at 45 CFR 164.514(a)-(c), is not PHI and is not subject to the Privacy Rule. The rule provides two methods of de-identification. The Safe Harbor method removes 18 specified identifiers (names, geographic subdivisions smaller than a state, dates, telephone numbers, fax numbers, email addresses, Social Security numbers, medical record numbers, health plan beneficiary numbers, account numbers, certificate or license numbers, vehicle identifiers, device identifiers, URLs, IP addresses, biometric identifiers, full-face photographs, and any other unique identifying number, characteristic, or code) and requires that the covered entity have no actual knowledge that the remaining data could be used to identify the individual. The Expert Determination method engages a qualified statistical expert who applies generally accepted statistical and scientific principles to determine that the risk of identification is very small.

The limited data set, defined at 45 CFR 164.514(e), is a middle position. It excludes most direct identifiers but permits dates, city, state, and ZIP code. It is not de-identified; it is still PHI for some purposes. Use of a limited data set requires a Data Use Agreement that obligates the recipient to use the data only for the agreed purpose, to apply appropriate safeguards, not to attempt re-identification, and to ensure that any subsequent recipients are bound by the same restrictions.

The minimum necessary standard at 45 CFR 164.502(b) requires that a covered entity make reasonable efforts to limit PHI to the minimum necessary to accomplish the intended purpose. The standard does not apply to disclosures to or requests by a healthcare provider for treatment, to disclosures to the individual, to uses or disclosures pursuant to authorization, or to uses or disclosures required by law. It does apply to most analytics. An analyst building a readmission model does not need patient names; the names are not minimum necessary for the model.

The HIPAA Security Rule, at 45 CFR Part 164 Subpart C, governs the safeguarding of electronic PHI. It requires administrative safeguards (security management process, workforce training, access management), physical safeguards (facility access controls, workstation security, device controls), and technical safeguards (access control, audit controls, integrity controls, transmission security). The CHDA exam tests recognition of the categories and the kinds of controls each requires, not detailed compliance configurations.

Audit logs are a Security Rule requirement and an analytic resource in their own right. Logs of who accessed which patient record, when, and from where can be analyzed to detect inappropriate access (snooping, identity theft) and to demonstrate compliance with the minimum-necessary standard. The 2019 OCR settlement with Anthem ($16 million, the largest HIPAA settlement at the time) was based in part on inadequate audit log monitoring that allowed an external breach to go undetected for nearly a year.

The Breach Notification Rule at 45 CFR Part 164 Subpart D requires notification to affected individuals, to the Secretary of HHS, and in some cases to media, when unsecured PHI is breached. The notification threshold is presumption of breach unless the covered entity can demonstrate through a risk assessment that there is a low probability that the PHI has been compromised. The risk assessment considers the nature and extent of the PHI involved, the unauthorized person who used or to whom the disclosure was made, whether the PHI was actually acquired or viewed, and the extent to which the risk has been mitigated. Notification must be made without unreasonable delay and in no case later than 60 days after discovery.

The HITECH Act of 2009 substantially expanded HIPAA's enforcement provisions and extended direct liability to business associates. It also established the meaningful use program that funded EHR adoption. The Cures Act of 2016 added the information-blocking framework and the API requirements discussed in Chapter 1. The interaction between HIPAA and the Cures Act has been a source of confusion: HIPAA is permissive (it permits but does not require many disclosures), while the Cures Act is restrictive of refusal to share (it prohibits practices that interfere with access except as excepted). A practice can be permitted by HIPAA and prohibited by the Cures Act. The CHDA exam expects candidates to recognize that compliance requires both rules to permit the action.

42 CFR Part 2 governs the confidentiality of substance use disorder records held by federally assisted programs. The rule is substantially more restrictive than HIPAA: it generally requires patient consent for any disclosure, even for treatment and payment, with limited exceptions. Recent revisions (the 2024 SAMHSA final rule, aligning Part 2 more closely with HIPAA for treatment, payment, and operations purposes) have softened some restrictions, but the rule still imposes higher protection for substance use disorder data than for general PHI. The CHDA candidate should recognize when a dataset is subject to Part 2 (records originating from a federally assisted substance use disorder treatment program) and treat it accordingly.

State privacy laws may impose additional restrictions, particularly around mental health records, HIV-related information, genetic information, and adolescent reproductive healthcare. The CHDA exam will not test detailed state-specific provisions but expects the candidate to recognize that state law may add to but not subtract from federal protections.

The Common Rule (45 CFR Part 46, also adopted by other federal agencies) governs human-subjects research conducted or funded by the federal government. It overlaps with but is distinct from HIPAA. A research project may need both IRB approval under the Common Rule and HIPAA authorization or waiver. The revised Common Rule (the "Revised Common Rule," effective in 2018) introduced changes including broad consent for secondary research use of identifiable private information, exemption categories for certain low-risk research, and single-IRB requirements for multi-site studies.

Exam Tip

TPO (treatment, payment, healthcare operations) is the category that covers most internal analytics. Quality improvement is operations; publication of findings turns the same work into research.

Exam Tip

The Safe Harbor de-identification method requires removal of 18 specific identifiers and is the simplest test on the exam. Expert Determination is the alternative when the Safe Harbor removals would render the data unusable for the intended purpose.

Exam Tip

A breach notification must be made within 60 days of discovery. The clock starts on discovery, not on the date the breach occurred.

Key Concept

TPO uses of PHI do not require authorization; research uses do, unless covered by an IRB waiver or another exception.

Key Concept

A limited data set is not de-identified and is still PHI for some purposes; its use requires a Data Use Agreement.

Key Concept

Minimum necessary is the operational test for every analytic disclosure of PHI except for treatment disclosures, individual disclosures, authorized disclosures, and required-by-law disclosures.

Key Concept

HIPAA permits but the Cures Act may prohibit refusal. Compliance requires both rules to permit the action.

0.18 Chapter Review Questions

Q1. A quality improvement team at a hospital is analyzing CAUTI (catheter-associated urinary tract infection) rates with the goal of reducing infections at the hospital. They do not plan to publish or generalize the findings. Which HIPAA category applies?

A) Research, requiring IRB approval or waiver.
B) Healthcare operations, permitted without patient authorization.
C) Marketing, requiring authorization.
D) Public health activity, requiring submission to CDC.

Answer: B — Internal quality improvement is healthcare operations under 45 CFR 164.501. The distinguishing feature from research is the absence of intent to generalize. Operations is a permitted use without authorization. If the team later decided to publish, the activity would shift to research and require additional review.

Q2. A dataset contains patient ZIP codes, dates of admission, and dates of discharge, but no names, addresses, or medical record numbers. Under the HIPAA Safe Harbor method, is the dataset de-identified?

A) Yes, because direct identifiers are removed.
B) No, because dates and ZIP codes are among the 18 identifiers requiring removal or aggregation.
C) Yes, but only if a Data Use Agreement is signed.
D) No, because the Safe Harbor method requires Expert Determination.

Answer: B — Safe Harbor de-identification at 45 CFR 164.514(b)(2) requires removal of all elements of dates (except year) and requires geographic subdivisions smaller than the state to be limited to the first three digits of the ZIP code only if combined population for that area is greater than 20,000. A dataset retaining full dates and full ZIP codes is not Safe Harbor de-identified; it is most likely a limited data set requiring a Data Use Agreement.

Q3. A breach is discovered on April 10. The investigation completes on May 15. Under the HIPAA Breach Notification Rule, by what date must affected individuals be notified?

A) Within 60 days of discovery — by June 9.

B) Within 60 days of investigation completion — by July 14.
C) Within 30 days of discovery — by May 10.
D) Within 90 days of discovery — by July 9.

Answer: A — The 60-day clock at 45 CFR 164.404(b) begins on the date of discovery, not on the date of investigation completion. Discovery is the first day the breach is known, or should have been known by exercising reasonable diligence. Delays through the investigation period do not toll the notification deadline.

Q4. A research request asks for a dataset including patient names, dates of birth, ZIP codes, diagnosis codes, and a flag indicating whether the patient received treatment for opioid use disorder at a federally assisted treatment program. Which legal framework applies in addition to HIPAA?

A) The Common Rule.
B) 42 CFR Part 2.
C) GINA (Genetic Information Nondiscrimination Act).
D) HITECH.

Answer: B — 42 CFR Part 2 governs the confidentiality of substance use disorder records originating from federally assisted treatment programs. Disclosure for research generally requires patient consent or a specific Part 2 exception, in addition to HIPAA compliance. The Common Rule applies to federally funded human-subjects research generally but is not specifically triggered by the substance use disorder element.

Q5. A health system refuses to provide a patient's records to a competing health system, even though the patient has requested the transfer, because the records contain analytics-derived risk scores that the health system considers proprietary. Which assessment is most accurate?

A) The refusal is permitted under the HIPAA Privacy Rule.
B) The refusal is permitted only if the patient consents.
C) The refusal likely constitutes information blocking under the Cures Act and is not within the eight defined exceptions.
D) The refusal is permitted because the data is proprietary.

Answer: C — HIPAA permits the disclosure (patient request, treatment exchange); the Cures Act prohibits refusal to share except under the eight defined exceptions, none of which cover commercial proprietary concerns. The interaction is exactly the scenario the Cures Act information-blocking framework was designed to address: a covered entity using "proprietary" or competitive arguments to withhold data that the patient has asked to be shared.

Clinical Classification Systems and Coding

Exam weight: approximately 7 percent

0.19 Learning Objectives

After completing this chapter, you will be able to:

- Identify the principal clinical classification and terminology systems used in U.S. healthcare and their purposes.
- Apply ICD-10-CM coding principles for diagnoses and ICD-10-PCS coding principles for inpatient procedures.
- Distinguish CPT and HCPCS Level II coding for outpatient services and supplies.
- Recognize the structure of MS-DRGs, APR-DRGs, APCs, and other groupers used for reimbursement and risk adjustment.
- Understand the role of SNOMED CT, LOINC, and RxNorm in clinical interoperability.

0.20 Content

Clinical classification underpins all healthcare analytics that involves diagnoses, procedures, medications, lab results, or any other coded clinical content. The CHDA candidate is not expected to be a credentialed coder, but is expected to understand the principal systems, what they encode, where they are used, and how they roll up into the groupers that drive reimbursement and risk adjustment.

ICD-10-CM (International Classification of Diseases, Tenth Revision, Clinical Modification) is the U.S. diagnosis coding system, maintained by the National Center for Health Statistics. It contains approximately 73,000 codes organized into 22 chapters. Codes range from three to seven characters. The first three characters represent the category; characters four through six provide etiology, anatomic site, and severity detail; the seventh character is an extension typically used for episodes of care for injuries, fractures, and pregnancies (initial encounter, subsequent encounter, sequela). The ICD-10-CM Official Guidelines for Coding and Reporting, jointly published by NCHS, CMS, AHA, and AHIMA, are updated annually and define the rules for selecting principal and secondary diagnoses, sequencing, and combination coding.

ICD-10-PCS (Procedure Coding System) is the U.S. inpatient procedure coding system, maintained by CMS. It contains over 78,000 codes, each exactly seven characters, with a uniform structure where each position has a specific meaning depending on the section. The Medical and Surgical section, the largest, uses sections labeled by body system, root operation (e.g., excision, resection, repair, replacement), body part, approach, device, and qualifier. ICD-10-PCS replaced ICD-9-CM Volume 3 in 2015 and was a substantial change in coding methodology — codes are constructed, not selected from a list. The CHDA candidate should know the seven-character structure and the concept of root operations, even without committing the code tables to memory.

CPT (Current Procedural Terminology), maintained by the American Medical Association, is the principal procedure code set for outpatient and physician services. It contains over 11,000 codes organized into three categories. Category I codes are the bulk of the system and cover common services (evaluation and management, surgery, radiology, pathology, medicine). Category II codes are optional performance measurement codes. Category III codes are temporary codes for emerging technology, services, and procedures. CPT is updated annually. CPT codes are five digits in Category I; some include modifiers indicating circumstances that affect the service.

HCPCS Level II codes, maintained by CMS, supplement CPT with codes for supplies, durable medical equipment, drugs administered by a method other than oral (J codes), and other items not covered by CPT. HCPCS Level II codes are five characters (one letter, four digits). The combination of CPT and HCPCS Level II is sometimes referred to as the HCPCS code set, with CPT designated as HCPCS Level I.

Medicare Severity Diagnosis Related Groups (MS-DRGs) are the inpatient prospective payment classification used by Medicare and many other payers. There are approximately 770 MS-DRGs. Each MS-DRG groups together inpatient encounters that are clinically similar and consume similar resources. Each DRG has a relative weight indicating its average resource intensity relative to the national average. Payment equals the DRG weight times the hospital's base rate, adjusted for geographic location and other factors.

Three categories of DRG payment exist within most major DRGs. The "without CC or MCC" version pays the base amount for an encounter without complications or comorbidities. The "with CC" version pays more for an encounter with at least one complication or comorbidity. The "with MCC" version pays the most for an encounter with at least one major complication or comorbidity. The CC and MCC lists are published by CMS and updated annually. Capturing CC and MCC conditions is a major focus of clinical documentation improvement because the difference between the three payment tiers can be thousands of dollars per case.

All Patient Refined DRGs (APR-DRGs), maintained by 3M, are a competing classification system used by many states for non-Medicare hospital reimbursement and by many quality reporting programs for risk adjustment. APR-DRGs include both a severity of illness (SOI) and risk of mortality (ROM) dimension, each with four levels (minor, moderate, major, extreme). The four-by-four structure produces 16 sub-DRGs for each base DRG, which provides finer-grained risk adjustment than MS-DRGs and is widely used in pediatric and obstetric populations where MS-DRGs perform less well.

Ambulatory Payment Classifications (APCs) are the outpatient prospective payment grouper for Medicare hospital outpatient services. Like DRGs, each APC has a relative weight, and payment is APC weight times the conversion factor. Outpatient encounters typically include multiple APCs (one per service), with packaging and discount rules applied to certain combinations.

Hierarchical Condition Categories (HCCs) are the Medicare Advantage risk adjustment grouper, maintained by CMS, that maps ICD-10-CM diagnoses to approximately 80 condition categories used to calculate a patient-level risk score. The risk score adjusts the capitated payment Medicare makes to MA plans, with higher-risk patients producing higher payments. HCCs are hierarchical in that, within related families, only the most severe category contributes (preventing double-counting of related conditions). HCCs are heavily emphasized in value-based contracting and in shared-savings programs because risk score accuracy directly affects financial performance.

SNOMED CT (Systematized Nomenclature of Medicine — Clinical Terms) is the comprehensive clinical terminology used worldwide for representing clinical content in EHRs. It contains more than 350,000 active concepts organized into a polyhierarchical structure with multiple parents per concept and explicit relationships (is-a, finding-site, causative-agent, etc.). SNOMED CT is the required terminology for problem lists in U.S. certified EHRs. Unlike ICD-10-CM, which is optimized for billing and statistical reporting, SNOMED CT is optimized for clinical specificity and computability.

LOINC (Logical Observation Identifiers Names and Codes) is the standard terminology for laboratory test results and clinical observations, maintained by the Regenstrief Institute. Each LOINC code has six parts: component (what is measured), property (mass concentration, presence, etc.), time aspect, system (specimen type), scale, and method. LOINC enables interoperable representation of lab results across systems with incompatible internal coding.

RxNorm is the standard terminology for medications, maintained by the National Library of Medicine. It provides normalized names for clinical drugs (generic plus strength plus dose form) and links them to commercial brand names and manufacturer-specific National Drug Codes (NDCs). RxNorm is the foundation of medication interoperability and decision support across systems.

The CHDA exam tests recognition of where each system fits in the analytic stack. Diagnosis analytics on inpatient claims uses ICD-10-CM. Procedure analytics on inpatient claims uses ICD-10-PCS. Outpatient procedure analytics uses CPT plus HCPCS Level II. Reimbursement analytics uses MS-DRGs, APR-DRGs, APCs, and HCCs depending on payer and program. Clinical analytics from EHR data uses SNOMED CT, LOINC, and RxNorm. A common exam scenario asks the candidate to identify the appropriate code system for a stated analytic purpose.

> **Exam Tip**
>
> The seventh character in ICD-10-CM codes is the encounter or episode extension. The exam may present a question hinging on the distinction between initial, subsequent, and sequela encounters.

> **Exam Tip**
>
> Within an MS-DRG family, the difference between "without CC/MCC," "with CC," and "with MCC" can substantially change payment. CDI programs target documentation of CC and MCC conditions.

> **Exam Tip**
>
> SNOMED CT is for clinical specificity; ICD-10-CM is for billing and statistical reporting. A scenario asking which to use for an EHR problem list is SNOMED CT.

> **Key Concept**
>
> ICD-10-CM has up to seven characters for diagnoses; ICD-10-PCS has exactly seven characters for inpatient procedures.

> **Key Concept**
>
> CPT covers outpatient and physician services; HCPCS Level II covers supplies, DME, and parenteral drugs.

> **Key Concept**
>
> MS-DRGs are CMS inpatient groupers; APR-DRGs are 3M's competing groupers used by many states and quality programs; APCs are CMS outpatient groupers; HCCs are CMS risk-adjustment groupers.

> **Key Concept**
>
> Interoperable clinical content uses SNOMED CT (concepts), LOINC (observations), and RxNorm (medications).

0.21 Chapter Review Questions

Q1. An analyst is building a quality measure on a Medicare Advantage population that requires calculating a patient-level risk score for prospective payment adjustment. Which classification system most directly drives the calculation?

A) ICD-10-PCS
B) MS-DRGs
C) HCCs
D) APR-DRGs

Answer: C — Hierarchical Condition Categories (HCCs) are the CMS risk-adjustment grouper used to calculate patient-level risk scores for Medicare Advantage capitated payments. Diagnoses recorded in ICD-10-CM map into HCCs, and the resulting risk score adjusts payment. MS-DRGs are inpatient prospective payment groupers; APR-DRGs are alternative inpatient groupers; ICD-10-PCS is a procedure code set.

Q2. Which classification system is the required terminology for problem lists in U.S. certified electronic health records?

A) ICD-10-CM
B) SNOMED CT
C) LOINC
D) HCPCS

Answer: B — The ONC certification criteria require SNOMED CT for problem list representation because of its clinical specificity and computability. ICD-10-CM is required for the billing problem list cross-walk but is not optimized for clinical use. LOINC covers laboratory and other observations; HCPCS covers procedures and supplies.

Q3. A code that includes the seventh character "A" most likely represents which kind of clinical scenario?

A) A sequela of an earlier condition.
B) An initial encounter for an injury.
C) A subsequent encounter for routine healing.
D) A planned readmission.

Answer: B — In ICD-10-CM, the seventh-character extension "A" typically indicates an initial encounter for an injury or external cause. "D" indicates a subsequent encounter for routine healing or recovery. "S" indicates a sequela. The exam may test these letter conventions even without requiring the candidate to identify the specific code.

Q4. An inpatient encounter for heart failure is documented without any complications or comorbidities. The encounter is assigned MS-DRG 293 (Heart Failure & Shock without CC/MCC). The patient's record includes a chronic condition that, if documented, would have qualified as a CC. What is the principal analytic consequence?
A) The hospital underbilled by failing to capture documented complexity, missing higher reimbursement.
B) The hospital overbilled and risks an audit.
C) No analytic consequence; the principal diagnosis drove DRG assignment.
D) The hospital must use APR-DRGs instead of MS-DRGs.

Answer: A — The case mix impact of CC capture is the textbook scenario for clinical documentation improvement. A documented CC moves the encounter from MS-DRG 293 (without CC/MCC) to MS-DRG 292 (with CC), producing a higher DRG weight and higher payment. The condition exists; documentation failure undervalues the hospital's compensable work.

Q5. Which code system would an analyst use to compare lab result patterns for hemoglobin A1c across two hospitals using different lab information systems?
A) ICD-10-CM
B) CPT
C) LOINC
D) RxNorm

Answer: C — LOINC provides standardized identifiers for laboratory observations including hemoglobin A1c. Internal lab system codes differ across hospitals; LOINC enables comparison. ICD-10-CM is for diagnoses, CPT for procedures, RxNorm for medications.

0.22 Practice Exam

The following 50 questions cover all seven domains proportionally and are intended to be completed under timed conditions (60 minutes target). Score yourself by domain after completion.

Q1. Which of the following best distinguishes data governance from data management?
A) Data governance is performed by IT; data management is performed by clinicians.
B) Data governance sets policy and accountability; data management executes operational handling of data.
C) Data governance is annual; data management is daily.
D) Data governance applies to PHI only; data management applies to all data.

Answer: B — Governance defines authority, accountability, and policy; management executes the operational handling. The split is conceptual, not by department or data type.

Q2. A patient changes legal name following a marriage. The patient dimension in the data warehouse currently uses Type 2 slowly changing dimensions. Which behavior is expected?
A) The old patient name is overwritten with the new name.
B) A new patient row is inserted with an effective_start date and the prior row's effective_end date is set; historical encounter joins reflect the name in effect at the time of service.
C) A new column is added to the patient table to store the prior name.
D) The patient record is duplicated under both names.

Answer: B — Type 2 SCD preserves history through dated versioned rows. Historical reporting joins on the version of the patient row active at the time of the encounter, producing point-in-time accuracy.

Q3. An analytic team produces a one-time scrub of duplicate patient records, reducing the duplicate rate from 4.2 percent to 0.8 percent. Six months later the rate has drifted to 3.1 percent. What is the most likely cause?
A) The scrub was technically defective.
B) Upstream registration processes that introduce duplicates were not addressed.
C) The EMPI algorithm was degraded.
D) The clean rate was not statistically achievable.

Answer: B — Data quality is sustained through upstream process improvement. A one-time cleanup without process change is consistently followed by regression as the registration processes that introduced the original duplicates continue to operate.

Q4. An O/E ratio of 1.12 with a 95 percent confidence interval of 1.04 to 1.21 indicates:
A) Better-than-expected performance, statistically significant.
B) Worse-than-expected performance, statistically significant.
C) Performance at expected, not statistically distinguishable.

D) Insufficient data to interpret.

Answer: B — O/E ratio greater than 1.0 indicates worse-than-expected performance. The 95 percent confidence interval excludes 1.0, so the difference is statistically significant.

Q5. A clinical decision support intervention powered by a predictive model is being deployed in an EHR. Under the ONC 2023 transparency rule, which documentation is required?

A) The vendor's licensing terms.
B) Information about the model's training data, intended use, validation, and performance characteristics, including any known limitations or risks.
C) The model's source code.
D) The model's pricing.

Answer: B — The ONC HTI-1 rule (Health Data, Technology, and Interoperability) requires source attributes and validation information for predictive decision support interventions in certified EHRs, including characteristics of training data, intended use, and known limitations.

Q6. A health system needs to share a dataset with an external researcher. The dataset includes admission and discharge dates and ZIP codes but no names, addresses, medical record numbers, or other direct identifiers. Which classification is correct?

A) De-identified under Safe Harbor.
B) Limited data set, requiring a Data Use Agreement.
C) Fully identified PHI, requiring authorization.
D) De-identified under Expert Determination.

Answer: B — Dates and ZIP codes are not removed in a limited data set but are removed under Safe Harbor de-identification. The dataset is a limited data set and requires a Data Use Agreement under 45 CFR 164.514(e).

Q7. The principal diagnosis on an inpatient discharge is the condition:

A) Most resource-intensive during the stay.
B) That, after study, occasioned the admission.
C) Listed first in the chart by the attending physician.
D) Most expensive to treat.

Answer: B — The Uniform Hospital Discharge Data Set (UHDDS) definition of principal diagnosis, codified by the ICD-10-CM Official Guidelines, is the condition established after study to be chiefly responsible for occasioning the admission. This is not necessarily the most resource-intensive or expensive condition during the stay.

Q8. Which chart type is best suited to displaying the distribution of patient ages in a cohort?

A) Pie chart.
B) Line chart.
C) Histogram.
D) Stacked bar chart.

Answer: C — A histogram displays the distribution of a continuous variable by binning values and showing frequency by bin. Pie charts show composition; line charts show trends; stacked bars show composition over time or category.

Q9. Under the HIPAA Breach Notification Rule, notification of affected individuals must be made within how many days of breach discovery?

A) 30 days
B) 60 days
C) 90 days
D) 180 days

Answer: B — The Breach Notification Rule at 45 CFR 164.404(b) requires notification without unreasonable delay and in no case later than 60 days after the discovery of the breach.

Q10. A coder reviews a chart in which the physician documented "pneumonia" without specifying the causative organism. Sputum culture in the chart shows Pseudomonas aeruginosa. Which CDI action is appropriate?

A) Code the more specific pneumonia code based on the culture result.
B) Issue a compliant query offering the physician a range of possible diagnoses including gram-negative pneumonia, Pseudomonas pneumonia, and "unable to determine."
C) Issue a query asking "Is this Pseudomonas pneumonia?"
D) Code unspecified pneumonia and move on.

Answer: B — Compliant queries offer multiple reasonable options drawn from the clinical evidence and avoid suggesting a single answer. A query naming only "Pseudomonas pneumonia" is leading. The coder should not assume the diagnosis from a culture result without physician documentation.

Q11. Which of the following best describes the c-statistic of 0.71 for a hospital readmission prediction model?

A) The model is wrong 71 percent of the time.
B) The model correctly classifies 71 percent of patients.
C) The model has 71 percent probability of ranking a randomly chosen positive case higher than a randomly chosen negative case.
D) The model's intercept is 0.71.

Answer: C — The c-statistic (area under the ROC curve) is the probability that the model assigns a higher predicted probability to a randomly chosen positive case than to a randomly chosen negative case. It is a measure of discrimination, not of accuracy.

Q12. A hospital's monthly readmission rate is reported as a line chart with the y-axis ranging from 12.5 percent to 14.0 percent. Which design defect is most directly visible?

A) Truncated y-axis exaggerates variation.
B) Line chart inappropriate for the data type.
C) Y-axis labels missing.
D) Color scheme inaccessible.

Answer: A — A tightly scaled y-axis that does not start at zero exaggerates the visual magnitude of variation. Tufte's graphical integrity principle calls for axis scales that do not distort the data.

Q13. An organization has policies on data access, technical enforcement of those policies, annual measurement of compliance, and active use of measurement results to drive process improvement. Which IGAM maturity level applies?

A) Level 2
B) Level 3
C) Level 4
D) Level 5

Answer: D — Level 5 corresponds to active use of measurement to drive continuous improvement. Level 4 is measurement without follow-through; Level 3 is documented enforcement; Level 2 is documented policy.

Q14. Which X12 transaction is used by a provider to inquire about a patient's eligibility and benefits with a payer?

A) 837
B) 835
C) 270
D) 278

Answer: C — The 270 transaction is the eligibility benefit inquiry; the 271 is the response. The 837 conveys claims; the 835 is the remittance advice; the 278 is referral and authorization.

Q15. A facility's gross mortality rate for a period equals:

A) Inpatient deaths divided by total admissions.
B) Inpatient deaths divided by total discharges (live discharges plus deaths).
C) Inpatient deaths divided by census.
D) Inpatient deaths divided by patient-days.

Answer: B — The gross mortality rate is inpatient deaths in the period divided by total discharges (live discharges plus deaths) in the period, often multiplied by 100 to express as a percentage.

Q16. An MS-DRG for heart failure has three payment tiers: without CC/MCC, with CC, and with MCC. Which abbreviation refers to a major complication or comorbidity?

A) MCC
B) CC
C) ROM
D) SOI

Answer: A — MCC is the major complication or comorbidity tier; CC is the (non-major) complication or comorbidity tier. ROM is risk of mortality (an APR-DRG concept); SOI is severity of illness (also APR-DRG).

Q17. Which terminology system is the U.S. standard for laboratory result interoperability?

A) SNOMED CT
B) ICD-10-CM

C) LOINC
D) RxNorm

Answer: C — LOINC is the standard terminology for laboratory observations and other clinical observations. SNOMED CT is for clinical concepts generally; ICD-10-CM for diagnoses; RxNorm for medications.

Q18. A request for the patient's full medical record is received from a provider treating the patient for an unrelated condition at another facility. Under HIPAA, this disclosure is:
A) Permitted under treatment as a TPO use.
B) Permitted only with patient authorization.
C) Permitted under the public health exception.
D) Prohibited without an IRB waiver.

Answer: A — Disclosures for treatment by another provider are permitted as a TPO use under 45 CFR 164.506. The minimum necessary standard does not apply to disclosures for treatment.

Q19. A research project proposes to use existing fully identified PHI without contacting patients for authorization. The IRB may waive authorization under 45 CFR 164.512(i) only if:
A) The research has potential commercial value.
B) The use involves no more than minimal risk, the research could not practicably be conducted without the waiver and without access to the PHI, and adequate plans for protection and destruction are in place.
C) The principal investigator holds a position at a covered entity.
D) The dataset is limited to the past three years.

Answer: B — The four criteria for an IRB or privacy board waiver of authorization are: no more than minimal risk to privacy; the research could not practicably be conducted without the waiver; the research could not practicably be conducted without the PHI; and adequate plans to protect the PHI and to destroy it when no longer needed.

Q20. Which of the following best describes the difference between Inmon's and Kimball's data warehouse approaches?
A) Inmon is bottom-up; Kimball is top-down.
B) Inmon is normalized and top-down; Kimball is dimensional and bottom-up using conformed dimensions.
C) Inmon is for cloud; Kimball is for on-premises.
D) There is no meaningful difference.

Answer: B — Inmon advocates building a comprehensive normalized enterprise warehouse first and then deriving dependent marts. Kimball builds dimensional marts directly and integrates them through conformed dimensions to form the enterprise warehouse.

Q21. A hospital's occupancy rate calculation requires which of the following inputs?
A) Total admissions and total discharges.
B) Inpatient service days, days in period, and bed complement.
C) Average length of stay and bed turnover.
D) Patient-days and patient-encounters.

Answer: B — Occupancy rate equals (inpatient service days / days in period) / bed complement, expressed as a percentage. The numerator (inpatient service days divided by days in period) is the average daily census.

Q22. Which of the following requires removal under the HIPAA Safe Harbor de-identification method?
A) The patient's birth year.
B) The patient's three-digit ZIP code prefix, if the combined population for that area exceeds 20,000.
C) The patient's full date of birth.
D) The patient's primary care provider type.

Answer: C — Safe Harbor requires removal of all elements of dates (except year) directly related to an individual. The first three digits of ZIP code may be retained if combined population exceeds 20,000. Provider type is not an identifier.

Q23. A new EHR vendor offers a population health module that exposes data via FHIR APIs. Which version of FHIR must be supported to meet current ONC certification requirements?
A) DSTU 2
B) STU 3
C) R4
D) R5

Answer: C — The ONC Cures Act Final Rule requires certified health IT to support standardized APIs based on FHIR R4. R5 is published but not yet a certification requirement as of 2026.

Q24. Which test would be most appropriate for comparing readmission rates between three payer categories?
A) Independent samples t-test.
B) Chi-square test of independence.
C) Paired t-test.
D) Pearson correlation.

Answer: B — Comparing categorical distributions (readmitted yes/no by payer category) is the chi-square scenario. The t-test compares means of continuous outcomes. A paired t-test compares matched continuous observations. Correlation describes relationships between continuous variables.

Q25. A data steward and a clinical leader disagree about whether to authorize an external vendor to access a patient list for outreach. Compliance is consulted. Which framework should compliance apply first?
A) Cures Act information-blocking rules.
B) Minimum necessary standard for the proposed disclosure, and identification of an applicable HIPAA permitted use or authorization.
C) The Common Rule.
D) State medical record retention statutes.

Answer: B — The threshold question for any external disclosure of PHI is whether a HIPAA permitted use applies or whether authorization is required, and whether the disclosure is limited to the minimum necessary. Information blocking is a separate analysis that may apply but is downstream of basic HIPAA permissibility.

Q26. Healthcare operations under HIPAA includes which of the following?
A) Marketing communications to patients about commercial products.
B) Sale of PHI to a third party.
C) Quality assessment and improvement activities, case management, and fraud and abuse detection.
D) Research designed to produce generalizable knowledge.

Answer: C — The definition of healthcare operations at 45 CFR 164.501 includes quality assessment, case management, fraud and abuse detection, and a list of related administrative activities. Marketing is separately regulated; research is not operations; sale of PHI is generally prohibited without authorization.

Q27. A patient overlay error in the EMPI most directly threatens:
A) Reporting accuracy only.
B) Patient safety, because clinical data from one patient may be applied to another at the point of care.
C) Billing efficiency only.
D) HIPAA Privacy Rule compliance only.

Answer: B — An overlay (two distinct patients merged into one enterprise record) is the most dangerous EMPI failure mode because at the point of care a clinician may see another patient's history mixed with the patient in front of them, leading to clinical decisions based on incorrect information.

Q28. A 5 percent missed charge rate on a hospital with $400 million in net patient revenue represents approximately:
A) $4 million in financial leakage.
B) $20 million in financial leakage.
C) $50 million in financial leakage.
D) Not enough information.

Answer: B — 5 percent of $400 million is $20 million. Missed charges convert directly to lost revenue when the encounter is otherwise billable. The CHDA candidate should be comfortable with this kind of order-of-magnitude estimation.

Q29. Which of the following is an extrinsic data quality characteristic?
A) Accuracy.
B) Consistency.
C) Timeliness.
D) Precision.

Answer: C — Timeliness depends on the fit between data availability and the use case, an extrinsic property. Accuracy, consistency, and precision are intrinsic properties of the data itself.

Q30. The principal advantage of a data lakehouse architecture over a traditional data lake is:
A) Lower cost of storage.
B) Support for ACID transactions, schema enforcement, and time travel queries on data-lake-format files.
C) Faster ingestion.
D) Built-in clinical analytics modules.

Answer: B — Lakehouse architectures (Delta Lake, Iceberg, Hudi) add transactional reliability, schema enforcement, and time travel queries to data lake storage. These features are the principal differentiation from generic data lakes.

Q31. Which of the following requires the longest retention under combined federal and typical state requirements for adult medical records?

A) 3 years
B) 5 years
C) 7 to 10 years
D) Permanent

Answer: C — Federal Medicare conditions of participation require five years; most state laws require seven to ten years for adult medical records. The longer requirement controls. Pediatric records typically require retention until the patient reaches majority plus a number of years.

Q32. A health system processes 837 claims data and 835 remittance data together to analyze denial rates by payer and reason code. Which CHDA-relevant analytic objective does this support?

A) Patient satisfaction measurement.
B) Revenue cycle performance improvement.
C) Clinical quality measurement.
D) Population risk stratification.

Answer: B — Denial rate analysis from paired 837/835 transactions is a core revenue cycle analytic pattern. The output drives process improvement in claims preparation, prior authorization, and documentation.

Q33. A statistical analysis finds a p-value of 0.001 for a 0.2 percentage point difference in mean length of stay between two hospitals. Which interpretation is most aligned with CHDA reporting principles?

A) The difference is statistically significant and operationally important.
B) The difference is statistically significant; operational importance depends on absolute magnitude and cost considerations.
C) The difference is not significant because the absolute size is small.
D) The result is too uncertain to report.

Answer: B — Statistical significance does not equal operational importance. A 0.2-day difference may matter in a high-volume hospital and not in a low-volume one. The CHDA candidate reports both the statistical and operational dimensions.

Q34. A clinical documentation improvement specialist writes a query asking "Was the patient's elevated creatinine due to acute kidney injury?" Which compliance assessment applies?

A) Compliant because it cites clinical evidence.
B) Non-compliant because it offers only one clinical possibility and is therefore leading.
C) Compliant because it asks the physician.
D) Non-compliant because creatinine is not a diagnostic finding.

Answer: B — A compliant query offers multiple reasonable options including the possibility that no specific diagnosis can be determined. This query is leading because it presents acute kidney injury as the only option.

Q35. Which standard is required for problem list interoperability in U.S. certified EHRs?

A) ICD-10-CM
B) SNOMED CT
C) RxNorm
D) ICD-10-PCS

Answer: B — Problem lists in certified EHRs must use SNOMED CT for clinical specificity. ICD-10-CM is used for cross-walked billing-relevant codes. RxNorm is for medications.

Q36. A dashboard for an operating room scheduler refreshes once per day at 06:00. The scheduler complains that mid-day cases that swap rooms are not reflected. Which design adjustment is most appropriate?

A) Increase the dashboard refresh frequency or implement a real-time view.
B) Add more historical data.
C) Replace bar charts with line charts.
D) Convert to a printed report.

Answer: A — The use case is operational and requires near-real-time signal. A daily refresh does not support mid-day room reassignment decisions. The dashboard cadence must match the action cadence.

Q37. A patient receives substance use disorder treatment at a federally assisted program. The treatment program later wants to share records with the patient's primary care provider for treatment coordination. Which legal framework imposes the most restrictive requirements?

A) HIPAA Privacy Rule alone.
B) 42 CFR Part 2, which historically requires patient consent for most disclosures including treatment.
C) The Cures Act.
D) State medical record laws.

Answer: B — 42 CFR Part 2 is the most restrictive applicable framework. Recent 2024 SAMHSA revisions have aligned Part 2 more closely with HIPAA for TPO purposes but the rule still requires patient-level protections substantially stronger than HIPAA's baseline.

Q38. Which of the following is a Type 2 slowly changing dimension implementation requirement?

A) Overwrite the old value with the new value.
B) Insert a new row with effective_start, effective_end, and current_flag fields preserving history.
C) Add a new column for the prior value.
D) Delete the prior row.

Answer: B — Type 2 preserves history through versioned rows with effective dating and a current-record flag. Historical reporting can reconstruct the value in effect at any historical date.

Q39. An analyst is asked to identify the most common reason for inpatient admission in a 12-month period. Which measure of central tendency is the appropriate summary?

A) Mean.
B) Median.
C) Mode.
D) Geometric mean.

Answer: C — The mode is the most frequent value and is the appropriate central tendency for categorical data. The most common admission reason is the mode of the principal diagnosis distribution. The mean and median apply to continuous data.

Q40. Which is true of the relationship between HIPAA and the Cures Act information-blocking rule?

A) HIPAA always overrides Cures Act requirements.
B) The Cures Act always overrides HIPAA requirements.
C) An action must be permitted by HIPAA and not constitute information blocking under the Cures Act; compliance requires both frameworks to permit the action.
D) The Cures Act applies only to vendors, not to providers.

Answer: C — HIPAA permits but does not require many disclosures; the Cures Act prohibits practices that interfere with access except under defined exceptions. An action may be permitted under HIPAA and still violate the Cures Act if a refusal to share is not within an exception. Both frameworks must permit the action.

Q41. A facility-level outcome report publishes a 23 percent readmission rate based on 17 cases. The published table suppresses the cell. Which is the most likely reason?

A) Statistical instability and re-identification risk in small cells.
B) The data was unavailable.
C) The hospital opted out of reporting.
D) The metric is not measured at the facility level.

Answer: A — Small-cell suppression in public reporting protects against both statistical instability (large confidence intervals on small samples) and re-identification risk (cells with few patients can identify specific individuals when combined with other public information). CMS typically suppresses cells with fewer than 11 patients.

Q42. A dataset is shared with a public health authority for surveillance of a reportable communicable disease. Under HIPAA, this disclosure is:

A) Permitted under the public health exception at 45 CFR 164.512(b).
B) Permitted only with patient authorization.
C) Prohibited without an IRB waiver.
D) Permitted only as de-identified data.

Answer: A — HIPAA permits disclosures to public health authorities authorized to receive such information for surveillance, investigation, and intervention. This is one of several "public interest" disclosures permitted without individual authorization.

Q43. Which classification system is the U.S. standard for inpatient hospital procedures (effective in inpatient settings)?

A) CPT
B) ICD-10-CM
C) ICD-10-PCS
D) HCPCS Level II

Answer: C — ICD-10-PCS is the U.S. inpatient procedure coding system, in use since 2015. CPT and HCPCS Level II are used for outpatient and physician services. ICD-10-CM is the diagnosis system.

Q44. A health system uses APR-DRGs for risk adjustment in its quality reporting. Which two dimensions are produced by APR-DRGs that MS-DRGs do not provide?

A) Length of stay and cost.
B) Severity of Illness (SOI) and Risk of Mortality (ROM), each with four levels.
C) Patient age and sex.
D) Principal and secondary diagnoses.

Answer: B — APR-DRGs assign each base DRG a 4-level Severity of Illness (SOI) and a 4-level Risk of Mortality (ROM), producing finer-grained risk adjustment than MS-DRGs. These dimensions are widely used in pediatric and obstetric populations.

Q45. A statistical model predicting 30-day readmission produces predicted probabilities ranging from 5 percent to 80 percent across the population. Among patients predicted at 30 percent, the observed rate is 50 percent. Which model property is most directly affected?

A) Discrimination.
B) Calibration.
C) Sensitivity.
D) Specificity.

Answer: B — Discrimination is the model's ability to rank cases; calibration is the alignment between predicted and observed probabilities. A model that systematically underpredicts in a probability band has a calibration problem, which matters more than discrimination for clinical decision support.

Q46. A facility's Case Mix Index has decreased from 1.82 to 1.71. Which of the following is the most clinically meaningful explanation?

A) Hospital acquired more high-acuity ICU capacity.
B) The hospital's case mix has shifted toward less complex cases, OR documentation has degraded, OR coding accuracy has declined.
C) The principal diagnosis distribution is unchanged.
D) Coders began capturing more comorbidities.

Answer: B — A CMI decrease has three principal candidate explanations: a real shift toward less complex cases, a documentation degradation that fails to capture complexity that is present, or a coding accuracy problem. Separating these three is a standard CDI analytic task.

Q47. The minimum necessary standard at 45 CFR 164.502(b) applies to:

A) All uses and disclosures of PHI.
B) All uses and disclosures except treatment, disclosure to the individual, authorized disclosures, and required-by-law disclosures.
C) Marketing uses only.
D) Research uses only.

Answer: B — Minimum necessary applies to most uses and disclosures but is exempted for treatment, disclosure to the patient, authorized disclosures, and required-by-law disclosures. Routine analytic disclosures are subject to the standard.

Q48. A reporting analyst notes that two operational dashboards show different counts of patients seen in a primary care clinic for the previous week. The first counts patients by encounter; the second counts unique patients (deduplicated). Which characteristic of data quality is most relevant to resolving the discrepancy?

A) Currency.
B) Definition.
C) Timeliness.
D) Granularity.

Answer: B — Both dashboards may be accurate against their own logic. The discrepancy reflects a definitional disagreement: encounters versus unique patients. Resolution is through the data steward and the data dictionary.

Q49. Which is the most appropriate use of a limited data set under HIPAA?
A) Public release for any purpose.
B) Research, public health, or healthcare operations purposes, under a Data Use Agreement.
C) Sale to third parties.
D) Direct patient outreach.

Answer: B — The limited data set at 45 CFR 164.514(e) may be used or disclosed for research, public health, or healthcare operations purposes, subject to a Data Use Agreement that imposes specific obligations on the recipient. Public release is not permitted.

Q50. A predictive model for diabetes risk is evaluated separately on Black and White patient subgroups. The c-statistic is 0.78 overall, 0.79 for White patients, and 0.62 for Black patients. Which response is most aligned with current CHDA principles on responsible analytics?
A) Deploy the model; overall discrimination is acceptable.
B) Document the subgroup performance gap, investigate causes (data representation, feature behavior, label noise), and consider remediation including retraining, calibration adjustment, or restricted deployment until the gap is closed.
C) Deploy the model only for White patients.
D) Discard the model entirely.

Answer: B — A meaningful subgroup performance gap is a recognized failure mode in healthcare predictive modeling. The CHDA-aligned response is to investigate, document, remediate, and disclose, not to deploy in the face of known disparate performance. Deploying only for one subgroup is a discriminatory action; discarding without analysis loses useful information.

Exam Quick Reference

Key Regulations

Regulation	Citation	Subject
HIPAA Privacy Rule	45 CFR Part 164 Subpart E	Use and disclosure of PHI
HIPAA Security Rule	45 CFR Part 164 Subpart C	Safeguarding of ePHI
HIPAA Breach Notification	45 CFR Part 164 Subpart D	60-day notification clock
Minimum Necessary	45 CFR 164.502(b)	Limit PHI to necessary amount
De-identification	45 CFR 164.514(a)-(c)	Safe Harbor and Expert Determination
Limited Data Set	45 CFR 164.514(e)	DUA-bound dataset
Research IRB Waiver	45 CFR 164.512(i)	Four-criteria waiver
Public Health Disclosure	45 CFR 164.512(b)	Surveillance and reporting
42 CFR Part 2	42 CFR Part 2	Substance use disorder records
Cures Act Final Rule	45 CFR Part 171	Information blocking; 8 exceptions
Common Rule	45 CFR Part 46	Human subjects research

Key Formulas

- Gross Mortality Rate = Inpatient Deaths / (Live Discharges + Deaths)
- Net Mortality Rate = (Inpatient Deaths − Deaths within 48 hr) / (Discharges − Deaths within 48 hr)
- Occupancy Rate = (Inpatient Service Days / Days in Period) / Bed Complement
- Average Daily Census = Inpatient Service Days / Days in Period
- Average Length of Stay = Total Discharge Days / Total Discharges
- Cesarean Rate = C-Section Deliveries / Total Deliveries
- Readmission Rate = Unplanned Readmissions within 30 Days / Index Discharges (risk-adjusted per CMS)
- Case Mix Index = Σ(DRG weights) / Number of Cases
- O/E Ratio = Observed Count / Expected Count from Risk Model

Statistical Tests

Test	Use
Independent t-test	Compare means of two independent groups
Paired t-test	Compare matched continuous observations
ANOVA	Compare means of three or more groups
Chi-square	Compare categorical distributions
Mann-Whitney U	Non-parametric two-group comparison
Linear regression	Continuous outcome on predictors
Logistic regression	Binary outcome on predictors
Time series (ARIMA)	Sequential observations over time

Code Systems Quick Map

System	Domain	Maintained by
ICD-10-CM	Diagnoses	NCHS
ICD-10-PCS	Inpatient procedures	CMS
CPT	Outpatient/physician procedures	AMA
HCPCS Level II	Supplies, DME, drugs	CMS
SNOMED CT	Clinical concepts	SNOMED International
LOINC	Lab/observation	Regenstrief Institute
RxNorm	Medications	NLM
MS-DRG	Inpatient grouping (Medicare)	CMS

System	Domain	Maintained by
APR-DRG	Inpatient grouping w/ SOI, ROM	3M
APC	Outpatient grouping (Medicare)	CMS
HCC	Risk adjustment (Medicare Advantage)	CMS

AHIMA Data Quality Characteristics (Ten)

Accuracy, Accessibility, Comprehensiveness, Consistency, Currency, Definition, Granularity, Precision, Relevancy, Timeliness.

IGAM Maturity Levels

Level	Description
1	Minimal or no formal governance
2	Developing: written policy exists
3	Defined: documented enforcement mechanisms
4	Managed: documented measurement of compliance
5	Transformational: continuous improvement from measurement

Glossary

APC (Ambulatory Payment Classification) — CMS outpatient prospective payment grouper.

APR-DRG — All Patient Refined Diagnosis Related Group, a 3M alternative grouper that includes Severity of Illness and Risk of Mortality dimensions.

Audit Log — A record of access events used to monitor for inappropriate access and demonstrate compliance.

Authorization — A patient's signed permission to use or disclose PHI for purposes beyond the permitted uses under HIPAA.

Business Associate — A person or entity that performs functions involving PHI on behalf of a covered entity.

c-statistic — Area under the ROC curve; a measure of predictive model discrimination (0.5 = chance, 1.0 = perfect).

Calibration — The alignment between predicted and observed event probabilities in a predictive model.

Case Mix Index (CMI) — Average DRG weight across a defined inpatient population.

CDI (Clinical Documentation Improvement) — A program that engages specialists to review documentation concurrently and query physicians for clarification.

Chi-square test — A statistical test comparing categorical distributions.

Common Rule — 45 CFR Part 46, the federal regulation governing human-subjects research.

Covered Entity — A health plan, healthcare clearinghouse, or healthcare provider that transmits PHI electronically; subject to HIPAA.

CPT — Current Procedural Terminology, maintained by the AMA, for outpatient and physician procedures.

Cures Act — The 21st Century Cures Act of 2016, the source of information-blocking regulation.

Data Custodian — IT personnel responsible for the technical security of data.

Data Dictionary — The authoritative record of every defined data element used in reporting.

Data Governance — The exercise of authority and control over data assets through policy.

Data Lake — Storage of raw data in object storage with schema-on-read.

Data Lakehouse — A modern architecture combining lake storage with warehouse-like transactional capabilities (Delta, Iceberg, Hudi).

Data Mart — A subject-area subset of a data warehouse.

Data Steward — The accountable owner of a data domain's definitions, quality, and authorized use.

Data Use Agreement (DUA) — Contract required for use of a limited data set under HIPAA.

Data Warehouse — A subject-oriented, integrated, time-variant, non-volatile data store for decision support.

De-identified Data — Data from which HIPAA-defined identifiers have been removed; not PHI.

DRG (Diagnosis Related Group) — A grouper that bundles similar inpatient cases for payment.

ELT — Extract, Load, Transform; modern variant of ETL.

EMPI (Enterprise Master Patient Index) — System that links source patient identifiers to a single enterprise identity.

ETL — Extract, Transform, Load; traditional integration pattern.

FHIR — Fast Healthcare Interoperability Resources, HL7's modern web-based standard (current required version R4).

HCC (Hierarchical Condition Categories) — CMS risk adjustment grouper used in Medicare Advantage.

HCPCS Level II — CMS code set for supplies, DME, and certain drugs.

HITECH Act — 2009 legislation expanding HIPAA enforcement and funding EHR adoption.

HL7 v2 — Legacy clinical messaging standard, pipe-delimited, still pervasive.

ICD-10-CM — U.S. diagnosis code set (up to seven characters).

ICD-10-PCS — U.S. inpatient procedure code set (exactly seven characters).

IGAM (Information Governance Adoption Model) — AHIMA framework with five maturity levels.

Information Blocking — Practices that interfere with the access, exchange, or use of electronic health information; prohibited except under eight defined exceptions.

Inmon Approach — Top-down normalized enterprise data warehouse with dependent marts.

IRB (Institutional Review Board) — Body that reviews research involving human subjects.

Kimball Approach — Bottom-up dimensional marts integrated through conformed dimensions.

Limited Data Set — Dataset excluding most direct identifiers but retaining dates and geographic information larger than street address; requires DUA.

Logistic Regression — Model of binary outcome as a function of predictors.
LOINC — Standard terminology for laboratory observations.
Mean / Median / Mode — Measures of central tendency.
Minimum Necessary — HIPAA standard requiring limitation of PHI to the minimum necessary for the purpose.
MS-DRG — Medicare Severity Diagnosis Related Group; the Medicare inpatient grouper.
Net Mortality Rate — Mortality rate excluding deaths within 48 hours of admission.
Observed-to-Expected (O/E) Ratio — Actual count divided by risk-adjusted expected count.
Overlay (EMPI) — Two distinct patients erroneously merged into one identity; dangerous failure mode.
PHI (Protected Health Information) — Individually identifiable health information held by a covered entity or business associate.
Predictive Analytics — Forecasting what is likely to happen.
Principal Diagnosis — The condition that, after study, occasioned the admission (UHDDS definition).
Prescriptive Analytics — Recommending what should be done.
RxNorm — Standard terminology for medications.
Safe Harbor De-identification — HIPAA method requiring removal of 18 specified identifiers.
SCD (Slowly Changing Dimension) — Dimensional modeling techniques for handling attribute change (Type 1 overwrite, Type 2 versioned rows, Type 3 prior-value column).
SNOMED CT — Comprehensive clinical terminology required for problem lists in certified EHRs.
Standard Deviation — Measure of dispersion around the mean.
Statistical Significance — Likelihood that an observed effect is not due to chance alone.
TPO (Treatment, Payment, Healthcare Operations) — HIPAA-permitted uses of PHI without authorization.
Uniform Hospital Discharge Data Set (UHDDS) — Definitional standard for hospital discharge reporting.
USCDI — United States Core Data for Interoperability; ONC-specified minimum data set for certified health IT.
X12 — EDI transaction standards required by HIPAA for administrative transactions (837 claims, 835 remittance, 270/271 eligibility, etc.).

Study Schedule

.1 Four-Week Plan (Recommended for Candidates with Active Clinical Data Analytics Experience)

Week 1: Foundations - Day 1: Read Chapter 1 (Data Governance). Complete review questions. - Day 2: Read Chapter 2 (Data Architecture). Complete review questions. - Day 3: Read Chapter 3 (Data Quality). Complete review questions. - Day 4: Re-review Chapters 1-3 weak points identified by review-question performance. - Day 5: Half-length practice (25 questions from Practice Exam). Score by domain. - Day 6: Read Appendix A and start Appendix B glossary review. - Day 7: Rest or light review.

Week 2: Analytics Deep Dive - Day 8: Read Chapter 4 first half (descriptive/diagnostic). Practice rate and ratio calculations. - Day 9: Read Chapter 4 second half (predictive/prescriptive). Practice O/E and c-statistic interpretation. - Day 10: Complete Chapter 4 review questions. Re-do any incorrect questions. - Day 11: Read Chapter 5 (Reporting and Visualization). Critique three dashboards in your own organization. - Day 12: Complete Chapter 5 review questions. - Day 13: Half-length practice (Practice Exam Q26-50). Score by domain. - Day 14: Rest.

Week 3: Compliance and Coding - Day 15: Read Chapter 6 (Compliance). Memorize key regulation citations. - Day 16: Complete Chapter 6 review questions. - Day 17: Read Chapter 7 (Coding). Build the code system quick-reference flashcards. - Day 18: Complete Chapter 7 review questions. - Day 19: Full Practice Exam under timed conditions (60 minutes). Score and analyze by domain. - Day 20: Targeted review of weakest domain. - Day 21: Rest.

Week 4: Consolidation - Day 22: Targeted review of second-weakest domain. - Day 23: Re-read all "Exam Tips" and "Key Concepts" across all chapters. - Day 24: Full Practice Exam re-take. Compare to Day 19. - Day 25: Final glossary pass. Make sure every term is known cold. - Day 26: Light review of Appendix A formulas. - Day 27: Rest or very light review. - Day 28: Exam day.

.2 Eight-Week Plan (Recommended for Career Transitioners or Those New to Healthcare Analytics)

Weeks 1-2: Governance and Architecture - Two weeks on Chapters 1 and 2 with supplemental reading on HIPAA, FHIR, and data warehousing.

Weeks 3-4: Quality and Analytics Foundations - Read Chapters 3 and 4 with extra time spent on statistical concepts. Work through rate and ratio calculations until the formulas are automatic.

Week 5: Reporting and Visualization - Chapter 5, with hands-on dashboard practice in a BI tool. Build at least one operational and one strategic dashboard from scratch.

Week 6: Compliance - Chapter 6, with supplemental reading on HIPAA, the Cures Act, and 42 CFR Part 2. Walk through the eight Cures Act information-blocking exceptions until they are memorized.

Week 7: Coding and First Full Practice Exam - Chapter 7. Build code-system flashcards. Full Practice Exam at the end of the week.

Week 8: Consolidation - Targeted review of weakest domains. Re-take the Practice Exam. Final glossary pass. Light review the day before the exam.

.3 Exam Day Logistics

- Confirm Pearson VUE appointment 48 hours in advance.
- Arrive 30 minutes early at a physical center; for online proctoring, complete the system check the day before.
- Bring two forms of identification (one government-issued photo ID required).
- For online proctoring, prepare a clean, well-lit, single-person room. No notes, no devices, no second monitor.
- Plan a 90-second-per-question pace; flag uncertain questions and return to them.

- Do not leave any question blank; there is no penalty for wrong answers.
- Eat a balanced meal beforehand; bring water if at a physical center (if permitted).
- Sleep adequately the night before. The exam is four hours of sustained concentration.

Good luck.

Consumer and Patient-Generated Health Data

.4 Learning Objectives

Upon completing this chapter, candidates will be able to:

- Distinguish among patient portals, personal health records, and third-party consumer health applications in terms of data ownership, access controls, and interoperability obligations.
- Explain the role of patient-reported outcomes and PRO performance measures in clinical quality programs and regulatory reporting.
- Describe how HL7 FHIR R4 and USCDI v3 standards govern the ingestion and exchange of wearable and remote patient monitoring data.
- Identify the principal data quality challenges specific to patient-generated health data and apply standard reconciliation strategies.
- Apply the information blocking rule, 21st Century Cures Act patient access provisions, and applicable privacy frameworks to consumer-generated health data scenarios.

.5 Patient Portals, PHR Systems, and Consumer Health Applications

Patient-generated health data (PGHD) encompasses any health-related data created, recorded, or gathered by patients and caregivers outside a clinical encounter. The three primary channels through which this data enters health information systems are patient portals, personal health record (PHR) systems, and consumer health applications.

Patient portals are provider-hosted, EHR-tethered web and mobile interfaces that give patients access to their own records. Under the 21st Century Cures Act (2016) and its implementing rules from ONC, covered entities operating patient portals must offer patients the ability to view, download, and transmit their health information at no cost. MyChart (Epic), FollowMyHealth, and athenahealth's patient portal are the dominant market implementations. These portals support bidirectional data exchange: patients can receive lab results, visit summaries, and care plans, and can submit symptom questionnaires, medication lists, and appointment requests that flow directly into the EHR workflow queue. Data submitted through a portal is attributed to the patient encounter and therefore subject to HIPAA's Minimum Necessary standard when accessed by workforce members.

Personal health records (PHRs) are patient-controlled repositories not hosted by a covered entity. Standalone PHR platforms such as Microsoft Health Vault (now retired) and current successors allow patients to aggregate data from multiple providers and devices. Because standalone PHRs operated by entities that are not covered entities or business associates fall outside HIPAA's direct jurisdiction, they are governed instead by the FTC Act's Section 5 unfair-or-deceptive-practices authority and, for commercial mobile health apps, by applicable FTC Health Breach Notification Rule requirements. This regulatory gap is a recurring CHDA exam focus.

Consumer health applications include Apple Health (HealthKit framework), Google Health Connect, Samsung Health, and a broad ecosystem of condition-specific apps (diabetes management, mental health trackers, fertility monitors). Apple Health aggregates data from device sensors, third-party apps, and, since iOS 11's Health Records feature, FHIR-formatted clinical documents from participating health systems. Google Health Connect (launched 2023, replacing Google Fit) uses a permissions framework that allows apps to read and write to a shared on-device data store. Both platforms implement FHIR R4 at their API layers for clinical data exchange, enabling structured data to be transmitted to EHR systems via SMART on FHIR authorization.

The critical distinction for exam purposes: a patient portal is a covered entity's interface, a standalone PHR is patient-controlled and frequently not HIPAA-covered, and a consumer app's regulatory status depends on whether the developer qualifies as a covered entity, business associate, or neither.

Exam Tip: The CHDA exam frequently tests whether a given scenario involves a HIPAA-covered entity. A fitness app sold directly to consumers by a non-healthcare company is NOT automatically a covered entity, even if it stores health data. The FTC — not OCR — is the primary enforcement authority for such apps.

.6 Patient-Reported Outcomes and PRO Performance Measures

Patient-reported outcomes (PROs) are measurements of any aspect of a patient's health status that come directly from the patient, without interpretation by a clinician. They may assess symptoms, functional status, health-related quality of life (HRQL), or treatment satisfaction. PROs are collected via standardized, validated instruments called patient-reported outcome measures (PROMs).

Established PROMs include the PROMIS (Patient-Reported Outcomes Measurement Information System) instruments developed by NIH, the EQ-5D for general health-related quality of life, the PHQ-9 for depression screening, and condition-specific tools such as the KOOS (Knee Injury and Osteoarthritis Outcome Score). PROMIS uses item response theory and computer adaptive testing (CAT), meaning the instrument selects follow-up questions dynamically based on prior answers, reducing patient burden while maintaining precision. This adaptive design means two patients may answer different questions yet receive comparable T-score-based results calibrated to the U.S. general population (mean 50, SD 10).

PRO performance measures (PRO-PMs) are a distinct and increasingly important category. A PRO-PM is a performance measure in which the data source is a PRO. The Centers for Medicare and Medicaid Services (CMS) incorporates PRO-PMs into the Merit-Based Incentive Payment System (MIPS) via the Quality Payment Program and into Hospital Outpatient Quality Reporting (OQR) and Inpatient Quality Reporting (IQR) programs. For example, the Total Hip Arthroplasty/Total Knee Arthroplasty (THA/TKA) functional status PRO-PM, adopted in the OQR program, requires hospitals to collect PROMIS-10 or HOOS JR / KOOS JR scores pre-operatively and at 12 months post-operatively. Reporting completeness thresholds apply: hospitals must achieve a minimum response rate (currently 60% for the voluntary reporting phase) or face public reporting impacts.

In clinical trials, PROs serve as primary or secondary endpoints under FDA guidance. FDA's 2009 PRO Guidance for Industry requires that PRO instruments used as trial endpoints demonstrate content validity (derived from patient input), construct validity, and reliability. FDA increasingly requires eCOA (electronic clinical outcome assessment) submission formats to ensure data integrity: time-stamping, audit trails, and prevention of batch data entry at sites.

For the health data analyst, PRO data management involves: instrument versioning control (different versions of PROMIS instruments are not interchangeable), missing data protocols (which imputation strategies are pre-specified in the analysis plan), and linkage to administrative claims or EHR data for risk adjustment. PRO data collected in routine care is lower quality than trial-collected data because patients may complete questionnaires in varied settings, assistance may be provided by family members, and administration timing may drift from protocol windows.

.7 Wearables, Remote Patient Monitoring, and FHIR-Based Ingestion

Wearable devices and remote patient monitoring (RPM) systems generate continuous or episodic physiologic data outside the clinical setting. Commercial wearables (Apple Watch, Fitbit, Garmin, Withings) capture steps, heart rate, heart rate variability, blood oxygen saturation (SpO2), skin temperature, ECG rhythm strips, and sleep stages. Clinical-grade RPM devices (iHealth, Biobeat, Dexcom continuous glucose monitors, Boston Scientific implanted cardiac monitors) capture higher-acuity data streams including interstitial glucose, blood pressure, weight, and cardiac rhythm with clinical precision standards.

Data formats differ by device class. Consumer wearables typically expose data through proprietary APIs (Apple HealthKit, Google Health Connect) before downstream conversion to HL7 FHIR. The FHIR Observation resource is the primary vehicle for transmitting PGHD: a single blood pressure reading maps to a FHIR Observation with code (LOINC 55284-4), value (systolic/diastolic components), subject (patient reference), effectiveDateTime, and device reference. Continuous glucose data maps to FHIR Observation with LOINC code 14745-4. Bulk time-series data from wearables may also use FHIR Bundle resources (batch or transaction type) to transmit multiple observations in a single API call.

USCDI v3 (U.S. Core Data for Interoperability, version 3, adopted in the 2023 ONC rule) explicitly includes patient-generated data elements. New USCDI v3 data classes relevant to PGHD include: Health Status/Assessments (functional status, mental/cognitive status, disability status, SDOH assessments), and the Patient Goals data element. Prior versions of USCDI did not enumerate PGHD as a discrete class; v3's inclusion creates an ONC-certified EHR obligation to capture and transmit these elements when present.

SMART on FHIR authorization enables third-party apps to request scoped, patient-authorized access to EHR data and to write PGHD back to the EHR. A patient using a diabetes management app can authorize it to write CGM readings to the EHR FHIR server using the FHIR write permission scope (`patient/Observation.write`). CMS Interoperability and Patient Access rules (CMS-9115-F, 2020) require payers to implement FHIR R4 Patient Access APIs, expanding the PGHD data flow context beyond providers.

RPM billing under CMS CPT codes 99453–99458 requires: an established patient-provider relationship, use of a medical-grade device, at least 16 days of readings per 30-day period for ongoing monitoring codes (99457/99458), and documentation of clinical staff review. Health data analysts support RPM programs by building dashboards that flag compliance gaps (patients below 16-day thresholds), alert clinicians to out-of-range values, and produce encounter documentation data.

.8 Data Quality Challenges in Patient-Generated Health Data

PGHD introduces data quality dimensions that differ substantially from clinician-generated EHR data. The four principal quality domains — completeness, accuracy, consistency, and timeliness — each manifest distinctively with patient-generated sources.

Completeness is the most frequently compromised dimension. Patients stop wearing devices, abandon portal questionnaires mid-session, or selectively report favorable readings. In RPM programs, non-adherence to device use is common among patients with the highest clinical burden — the same population whose data is most needed for risk stratification. Analysts must distinguish missing-at-random from missing-not-at-random patterns, because the latter introduces systematic bias in downstream analytics. A patient who stops recording blood pressure readings because values are alarming is a missing-not-at-random pattern that biases summary statistics toward falsely normal distributions.

Accuracy errors in PGHD arise from three sources: device measurement error, patient input error, and transcription error at portal entry. Consumer-grade blood pressure cuffs may have systematic calibration offsets. Patients entering medication lists manually in portals introduce spelling errors (drug name misspellings), wrong dosage units, and duplicate entries under brand and generic names. Patients may enter weight in kilograms when the field expects pounds, producing implausible outliers (a patient appears to weigh 165 lbs one day and 165 kg the next after unit confusion).

Duplicate record reconciliation is a specific accuracy problem at the EHR-PGHD boundary. When a patient's Apple Health record pushes immunizations to an EHR that already contains those records from a prior provider, the EHR must deduplicate without discarding legitimate variations. The FHIR `$match` operation and probabilistic matching algorithms (using date, code, performer, and patient demographic identifiers) are standard technical approaches. False positive deduplication — merging records that are not truly the same — can delete valid clinical events.

Consistency problems emerge when the same data element is captured redundantly across portal, app, and EHR channels. A patient's smoking status entered as "former smoker, quit 2019" in Apple Health may conflict with "current smoker" in the EHR from a prior visit. Conflict resolution logic must be version-controlled and documented: last-write-wins policies are inappropriate for clinical data because recency does not equal accuracy.

Exam Tip: For CHDA exam scenarios involving PGHD quality, remember that the analyst's role includes defining provenance metadata — recording the source (patient self-report, consumer device, clinical device) in the data dictionary. Data without documented provenance cannot be reliably used in quality measures or research. Provenance is captured in FHIR using the Provenance resource linked to Observation resources.

Timeliness problems include delayed submission (patients entering a week of readings in one session, back-dating entries) and clock drift on consumer devices. FHIR Observation resources carry both `effectiveDateTime` (the time the measurement occurred) and `issued` (when it was recorded in the system); a large gap between these fields signals retrospective entry and reduces data reliability for time-sensitive clinical decisions.

.9 Regulatory Context — 21st Century Cures Act, Information Blocking, and App Developer Obligations

The 21st Century Cures Act (P.L. 114-255, 2016) and ONC's implementing regulations (21st Century Cures Act Final Rule, 2020; 45 CFR Part 170) establish the primary federal regulatory framework for patient access to health data, including PGHD.

Patient access requirements under the Cures Act mandate that ONC-certified health IT modules support patient electronic access to their health information without special effort. The API requirements (45 CFR 170.315(g)(10)) require certified EHR systems to implement FHIR R4-based APIs that allow patients to authorize third-party applications to receive their health data. Health systems must make all data classes and elements in the USCDI available through these APIs. The requirement is technology-neutral with respect to the receiving app, but the certified API must conform to the SMART on FHIR authorization framework.

The information blocking rule (45 CFR Part 171) prohibits covered actors — health IT developers, health information networks/exchanges, and healthcare providers — from practices that unreasonably interfere with the access, exchange, or use of electronic health information (EHI). For PGHD contexts, this means a health system cannot block a patient's authorized app from receiving PGHD that the health system holds (e.g., portal-submitted questionnaires stored in the EHR). Eight regulatory exceptions define permitted restrictions: the Preventing Harm exception (withholding data for safety reasons), the Privacy exception (withholding based on applicable law), the Security exception, the Infeasibility exception, the Health IT Performance exception, the Content and Manner exception, the Fees exception, and the Licensing exception. Penalties for information blocking by providers can reach $1 million per violation under CMS's Conditions of Participation enforcement.

App developer obligations depend on how the developer is classified. A developer that creates a patient-facing app but is not a covered entity or business associate is outside HIPAA's direct reach. However: - The FTC Health Breach Notification Rule (amended 2023) requires PHR-related app vendors to notify consumers, the FTC, and media of unauthorized acquisition of identifiable health information. The 2023 amendments explicitly extended coverage to health apps that draw data from non-covered entity sources. - ONC-certified health IT developers are subject to the information blocking prohibitions as covered actors. - Developers accessing EHR data through SMART on FHIR APIs must comply with the API terms of service set by the EHR vendor and any contractual data-use restrictions imposed by the health system.

The Cures Act also created the Trusted Exchange Framework and Common Agreement (TEFCA), a voluntary national framework for health information exchange. TEFCA's Qualified Health Information Networks (QHINs) are required to support individual access services (IAS), enabling patients to request their records from any QHIN participant — including records containing PGHD stored in a QHIN-connected system.

Exam Tip: The CHDA exam distinguishes between ONC and CMS regulatory authority. ONC governs health IT certification and information blocking. CMS governs interoperability requirements for payers and providers as conditions of Medicare/Medicaid participation. Both issued rules implementing Cures Act mandates but through separate regulatory pathways and enforcement mechanisms.

.10 Privacy and Consent for Consumer-Generated Data — Secondary Use, De-identification, and Third-Party Data Flows

Consumer-generated health data raises privacy challenges that differ from traditional clinical data governance because the data originates outside covered entity systems, is often governed by app terms of service rather than HIPAA, and is subject to secondary use in ways patients may not anticipate.

Secondary use refers to using health data for purposes beyond the primary purpose for which it was collected. PGHD collected by a fitness app to help a user track exercise steps may be secondarily used by the app developer for advertising targeting, actuarial modeling, or sale to data brokers. Under HIPAA, secondary use of PHI by covered entities requires either patient authorization or an applicable exception (treatment, payment, operations, public health, research with IRB waiver). Consumer apps operating outside HIPAA use terms-of-service agreements to obtain consent for secondary use, but research shows that fewer than 10% of users read privacy policies and that comprehension of data sharing practices is low even among health-literate users.

De-identification of PGHD for secondary use follows the same two methods defined at 45 CFR 164.514(b) as apply to EHR data, but with important practical complications. The Safe Harbor method requires removal of 18 specified identifiers; for consumer device data, quasi-identifiers including step-count patterns, sleep timing, and GPS-derived home location can re-identify individuals even after Safe Harbor de-identification. The Expert Determination method requires a qualified statistician to certify that re-identification risk is very small — a higher bar that is appropriate when PGHD will be aggregated and shared externally. Geolocation data embedded in wearable records is particularly re-identification-prone and should be stripped at the field level before de-identified datasets are shared.

Third-party data flows in consumer health ecosystems are complex. A patient authorizes App A to read from Apple Health, which itself aggregates from App B (a CGM), App C (a pharmacy app), and App D (a mental health journaling app). App A may share derived insights with a data partner under its privacy policy. The patient's consent to Apple Health's terms does not automatically constitute consent for App A to share with that data partner. Each app-to-app data sharing relationship has its own consent and regulatory posture.

FHIR-based data flows introduce additional governance considerations. When a patient authorizes a SMART on FHIR app to pull their EHR data, the covered entity transmitting the data transfers regulatory accountability to the app once the data leaves the covered entity's system. ONC guidance clarifies that covered entities are not liable for what HIPAA-exempt apps do with data they receive through authorized patient-directed sharing under 45 CFR 164.524. This is the "patient-directed disclosure" doctrine: when a patient directs their own data to a third party, the covered entity's obligation ends at transmission.

Consent models for research use of PGHD include broad consent (45 CFR 46.116(d), added by 2018 Common Rule revisions), which allows patients to consent once to future unspecified research on biospecimens and health data under defined limitations. Broad consent is increasingly used for EHR-embedded research registries that collect PRO data longitudinally. Dynamic consent platforms — digital interfaces that allow patients to modify research participation permissions in real time — are emerging but not yet standardized across institutions.

State law complicates PGHD governance. Washington State's My Health MY Data Act (2023) extends health data protections to consumer apps regardless of HIPAA coverage status, requiring geofenced consent before collecting location data for health inferences and prohibiting certain secondary uses. California's CMIA (Confidentiality of Medical Information Act) extends to certain health app data. Health data analysts managing multi-state data assets must maintain a jurisdiction matrix tracking applicable state laws for each data source.

.11 Key Concepts

- **Patient portal vs. standalone PHR regulatory status:** Patient portals operated by covered entities are HIPAA-covered; standalone PHRs operated by non-covered entities are regulated primarily by the FTC, not OCR.
- **USCDI v3 PGHD data classes:** Version 3 adds Health Status/Assessments (functional, mental/cognitive, disability status, SDOH) and Patient Goals as discrete data elements that certified EHRs must support.
- **FHIR Observation resource:** The primary FHIR resource used to transmit PGHD including wearable readings; contains LOINC-coded data element, value, effectiveDateTime, subject, and optional device reference.
- **PROMIS T-score calibration:** PROMIS instruments are calibrated to the U.S. general population with mean 50, standard deviation 10; higher scores indicate more of the measured concept (higher pain = more pain, higher physical function = better function — direction varies by domain).
- **Information blocking eight exceptions:** Preventing Harm, Privacy, Security, Infeasibility, Health IT Performance, Content and Manner, Fees, and Licensing — all are affirmative defenses; the actor must satisfy exception criteria to avoid liability.
- **RPM billing minimum threshold:** CMS requires at least 16 days of remote physiologic monitoring data per 30-day period to bill CPT 99457 (20 or more minutes of clinical staff time) and 99458 (each additional 20 minutes).
- **FTC Health Breach Notification Rule (2023):** Amended to explicitly cover health apps that are not HIPAA-covered entities, requiring consumer notification, FTC notification, and (if >500 affected) media notification within 60 calendar days of discovering a breach.
- **Patient-directed disclosure doctrine:** Under 45 CFR 164.524, when a patient directs their covered entity to transmit records to a third-party app, the covered entity bears no HIPAA liability for the app's subsequent use of that data.

.12 Review Questions

1. A patient uses a commercially available fitness tracking app (not affiliated with any health system) to log daily steps and sleep duration. The app's privacy policy permits sharing de-identified usage data with advertising partners. Under which regulatory framework does OCR have primary enforcement jurisdiction over the app developer's data practices?

A. HIPAA Privacy Rule
B. FTC Act Section 5
C. 21st Century Cures Act information blocking rule
D. HITECH Act Breach Notification Rule

Correct Answer: B.

The app developer is not a covered entity or business associate under HIPAA, so OCR has no jurisdiction. The FTC Act Section 5, which prohibits unfair or deceptive trade practices, is the primary federal authority over non-HIPAA health app developers. The information blocking rule applies to health IT developers of ONC-certified products, healthcare providers, and health information networks — not to general consumer fitness apps. The HITECH Breach Notification Rule applies to covered entities and their business associates; the FTC Health Breach Notification Rule (not HITECH) would apply to a PHR-related app.

2. A health system's EHR receives a FHIR Bundle from a patient's Apple Health app containing 14 days of blood pressure readings. The analyst notices that the `issued` timestamp on each Observation is the same date, while the `effectiveDateTime` values span 14 different days. What data quality issue does this pattern indicate?

A. Duplicate record submission
B. Retrospective batch entry of readings
C. Device clock drift requiring recalibration
D. FHIR version incompatibility between sender and receiver

Correct Answer: B.

When `issued` (recording time) is a single date but `effectiveDateTime` (measurement time) spans multiple past dates, the pattern indicates that the patient entered all readings at once rather than at the time of measurement. This is retrospective batch entry, which reduces data reliability for time-sensitive clinical decisions because the readings were not contemporaneous. Device clock drift would produce small, systematic offsets across all timestamps rather than a single `issued` date. Duplicate submission would produce repeated identical Observations. FHIR version incompatibility would likely produce parsing errors, not this timestamp pattern.

3. Under USCDI v3, which of the following data classes was newly added to the required interoperability framework specifically to address patient-generated health data?

A. Allergies and Intolerances
B. Laboratory
C. Health Status/Assessments
D. Immunizations

Correct Answer: C.

USCDI v3, adopted in the 2023 ONC rule, added Health Status/Assessments as a new data class, which includes functional status, mental/cognitive status, disability status, and SDOH assessments — elements that are primarily patient-generated or patient-reported. Allergies and Intolerances, Laboratory, and Immunizations were present in earlier USCDI versions. Health Status/Assessments was not enumerated as a discrete data class in USCDI v1 or v2, making its v3 inclusion the key regulatory change extending interoperability obligations to PGHD.

4. A hospital is required to collect PROMIS-10 Global Health scores from total knee arthroplasty patients pre-operatively and at 12 months for the CMS OQR PRO-PM program. The hospital achieves a 55% response rate at 12 months. What is the most likely regulatory consequence?

A. Immediate financial penalty assessed by CMS
B. The hospital's data is excluded from the national benchmark
C. Public reporting impacts may result if the threshold is not met in the reporting period
D. The hospital must submit amended data using HOOS JR instead of PROMIS-10

Correct Answer: C.

CMS OQR PRO-PMs operate under a voluntary reporting phase with a minimum response rate threshold (currently 60%). Hospitals that do not meet the threshold may face public reporting impacts — their data may be publicly reported as below minimum threshold rather than as a calculated performance rate. There is no immediate financial penalty structure for the PRO-PM collection itself under the current voluntary phase. The national benchmark continues regardless of individual hospital response rates. PROMIS-10 and HOOS JR are both accepted instruments for the TKA PRO-PM; the hospital does not need to switch instruments based on response rate.

5. A covered entity transmits a patient's complete medical record — including portal-submitted PRO questionnaire data — to a third-party SMART on FHIR app at the patient's explicit direction. The app subsequently sells the patient's mental health PRO scores to a data broker. Under ONC guidance, who bears HIPAA liability for the data broker transaction?

A. The covered entity that transmitted the data
B. The SMART on FHIR app developer
C. Both the covered entity and the app developer jointly
D. Neither, because HIPAA does not apply once data leaves the covered entity

Correct Answer: B.

Under the patient-directed disclosure doctrine (45 CFR 164.524), when a covered entity transmits records to a third-party app at the patient's direction, the covered entity's HIPAA obligation ends at transmission. However, if the SMART on FHIR app developer is itself a covered entity or business associate, it retains HIPAA obligations. If the app developer is not a covered entity, HIPAA does not directly apply to the developer's subsequent disclosure — but the developer may face FTC enforcement. The covered entity is not jointly liable for what the app does after receiving patient-directed data. Answer D is partially correct but incomplete: HIPAA still applies to HIPAA-covered recipients of the data.

6. Which FHIR resource is used to document the source and chain of custody of a PGHD observation transmitted from a wearable device to an EHR?

A. Observation
B. Device
C. Provenance
D. AuditEvent

Correct Answer: C.

The FHIR Provenance resource is specifically designed to record the source, author, and chain of custody for other FHIR resources. When a wearable device observation is transmitted to an EHR, a linked Provenance resource documents that the observation originated from the patient's device, when it was recorded, and what agent (patient, app, device) created it. The Observation resource holds the measurement value and metadata but does not itself carry source chain-of-custody documentation. Device resource describes the device's characteristics. AuditEvent records security-relevant system events (access, disclosure) rather than data provenance.

7. A clinical researcher wants to use PROMIS-29 data collected during routine outpatient visits for a new observational study. The IRB approved a broad consent protocol under 45 CFR 46.116(d). Which condition is REQUIRED for broad consent to be valid for this future research use?

A. Patients must re-consent for each specific study using the PRO data
B. Broad consent must include a description of the types of research that may be conducted
C. Broad consent is not applicable to health data; only biospecimens qualify
D. The researcher must de-identify all PRO data before use under broad consent

Correct Answer: B.

The 2018 Common Rule revisions at 45 CFR 46.116(d) established broad consent as a valid mechanism for future research on stored identifiable biospecimens and identifiable private information (including health data, not just biospecimens). For broad consent to be valid, it must describe, among other elements, the types or categories of research that may be conducted — even if the specific studies are not yet defined. Patients are not required to re-consent for each study if broad consent criteria are satisfied. De-identification of data before use is not a requirement of broad consent; it is a separate pathway (exemption category 4) to avoid IRB review.

8. A health data analyst is evaluating the completeness of RPM blood pressure data for a hypertension management program. She finds that patients with the worst blood pressure control have significantly more missing readings than well-controlled patients. Which type of missingness mechanism does this represent, and how does it affect analysis validity?

A. Missing completely at random (MCAR); no systematic bias is introduced
B. Missing at random (MAR); bias can be corrected through covariate adjustment
C. Missing not at random (MNAR); missingness is related to the unobserved value itself, introducing systematic bias
D. Structural missingness; it reflects correct absence of data for non-qualifying periods

Correct Answer: C.

When patients with worse blood pressure control are more likely to have missing readings — because high values may prompt them to avoid recording — the missingness mechanism is Missing Not at Random (MNAR). The probability of missingness depends on the unobserved value itself, not just on observed covariates. This introduces systematic bias: summary statistics and outcomes analyses will be biased toward falsely favorable blood pressure distributions. MCAR would require the probability of missingness to be independent of any data values. MAR would allow bias correction through observed covariates, but MNAR cannot be fully corrected through standard imputation methods. Structural missingness refers to logically impossible data (e.g., post-discharge readings for a deceased patient).

9. Under the 21st Century Cures Act information blocking rule, which of the following exceptions would permit a health system to restrict a patient's authorized app from receiving sensitive mental health notes stored in the EHR?

A. The Fees exception
B. The Licensing exception
C. The Privacy exception
D. The Content and Manner exception

Correct Answer: C.

The Privacy exception (45 CFR 171.202) permits a covered actor to limit access or exchange of EHI to the extent necessary to protect patient privacy under applicable federal or state law. If a state's mental health confidentiality statute restricts disclosure of psychotherapy notes without specific written authorization that exceeds standard HIPAA authorization, the health system may invoke the Privacy exception to withhold those records from an app that has not obtained the requisite authorization. The Fees exception governs pricing for access. The Licensing exception governs technology licensing restrictions. The Content and Manner exception permits a covered actor to limit the manner of fulfilling a request if it cannot satisfy the preferred manner and is offering a reasonable alternative.

10. A health system's data governance team is designing a de-identification protocol for PGHD that includes continuous glucose monitoring (CGM) readings and step-count time series. They are using the Expert Determination method. Which factor most distinguishes Expert Determination from the Safe Harbor method for this use case?

A. Expert Determination does not require removal of the 18 HIPAA-specified identifiers
B. Expert Determination requires a qualified statistician to certify that re-identification risk is very small given anticipated recipients and data uses
C. Expert Determination is only valid for research; Safe Harbor is required for operational analytics
D. Expert Determination requires IRB approval before de-identified data can be shared

Correct Answer: B.

The Expert Determination method (45 CFR 164.514(b)(1)) requires a person with appropriate knowledge and experience in statistical and scientific principles to apply those principles and certify that the risk of identifying an individual is very small, given the anticipated recipients and uses of the data. For CGM and step-count time series — which are highly re-identifying due to behavioral patterns — Expert Determination is preferable because it explicitly addresses the actual re-identification risk profile of the specific dataset. Safe Harbor requires removal of 18 enumerated identifiers but does not require a formal risk assessment; it may underprotect complex time-series data. Expert Determination is not restricted to research contexts, and it does not require IRB approval (IRB review governs human subjects research, not de-identification methods per se).

Health Data Interoperability and Exchange

Learning Objectives

- Explain the HL7 FHIR R4 and R5 resource model, RESTful interaction patterns, and SMART on FHIR authorization scopes used in patient-facing and provider-facing applications.
- Describe the evolution of USCDI across versions 1, 2, and 3, identifying the data classes and elements added at each version and their regulatory significance.
- Interpret US Core Implementation Guide conformance language, distinguishing must-support obligations from optional elements and explaining how profiles constrain base FHIR resources.
- Compare C-CDA document types — Continuity of Care Document, Discharge Summary, and Referral Note — according to their clinical trigger events and required data sections.
- Summarize the ONC 21st Century Cures Act Final Rule API mandates, including patient access, provider access, and payer-to-payer exchange requirements and associated compliance timelines.

.13 HL7 FHIR R4/R5: Resource Model, RESTful API, and SMART on FHIR

HL7 Fast Healthcare Interoperability Resources (FHIR) is a modern health data standard published by Health Level Seven International. FHIR organizes clinical and administrative data into discrete, web-native units called resources. Each resource represents a single clinical concept: a Patient resource holds demographics and identifiers; a Condition resource holds a diagnosis with onset date, clinical status, and coded representation; an Observation resource holds a lab result, vital sign, or survey response paired with its value and status. Resources reference one another using logical identifiers rather than embedding nested content, keeping payloads compact and modular.

FHIR R4, finalized in 2019, is the version mandated by the ONC 21st Century Cures Act Final Rule and is therefore the version most heavily tested on certification examinations. R5, published in 2023, introduced subscriptions via topic-based channels, refined the Appointment and Schedule resources, and strengthened support for clinical decision support hooks, but regulatory mandates as of 2026 still cite R4 as the minimum conformance target.

Every FHIR server exposes a RESTful API anchored to a base URL called the service base. The standard defines five core HTTP interactions: READ retrieves a single resource by logical ID; SEARCH returns a Bundle of matching resources filtered by query parameters; CREATE posts a new resource and returns a server-assigned ID; UPDATE replaces an existing resource; DELETE removes it. A conformant server publishes a CapabilityStatement resource at the path /metadata, declaring which resource types it supports, which interactions it allows, and which search parameters it recognizes. The CapabilityStatement is the machine-readable contract between client and server.

SMART on FHIR, developed at Boston Children's Hospital and now an HL7 standard, layers OAuth 2.0 authorization on top of FHIR REST. It defines two launch contexts: the standalone launch, in which an app launches outside an EHR and authenticates directly against an authorization server, and the EHR launch, in which the EHR passes a launch token to the app at startup so the app can request context (current patient, current encounter) without prompting the user. Scopes in SMART on FHIR follow the pattern patient/[ResourceType].[read|write|*] for patient-context access and user/[ResourceType].[read|write|*] for practitioner-context access. The scope openid profile enables the app to retrieve a user identity token. Apps must request only the minimum scopes needed (principle of least privilege), and authorization servers may grant a narrower scope than requested.

Exam Tip: On the CHDA exam, distinguish between FHIR R4 (the regulatory-mandated version under ONC rules) and R5 (the current published version). Questions about API mandate compliance always refer to R4 unless the question explicitly states otherwise.

.14 USCDI Versions 1, 2, and 3: Data Classes and Required Elements

The United States Core Data for Interoperability (USCDI) is a standardized set of health data classes and constituent data elements that must be supported across certified health IT systems. ONC manages USCDI and publishes new versions on an annual cadence, advancing elements through a public comment and priority-ranking process before promotion to a new version.

USCDI v1, incorporated into the ONC 21st Century Cures Act Final Rule (85 FR 25642, May 2020), established the baseline. It defined 12 data classes: Allergies and Intolerances, Assessment and Plan of Treatment, Care Team Members, Clinical Notes, Goals, Health Concerns, Immunizations, Laboratory, Medications, Patient Demographics, Problems, Procedures, Provenance, Smoking Status, Unique Device Identifiers for Implantable Devices, and Vital Signs. Each class contains data elements at a level of granularity specific enough to drive system implementation. For example, the Patient Demographics class includes first name, last name, previous name, sex (not gender), date of birth, address, phone number, and communication preferences as distinct elements.

USCDI v2, finalized in July 2021, expanded the standard with seven new data classes and additional elements within existing classes. New classes included Diagnostic Imaging, Encounter Information, Health Status/Assessments (encompassing functional status and disability status), Pediatric Vital Signs, Patient-Reported Data (Patient-generated health data and social determinants of health screenings), Pregnancy Status, and Sexual Orientation and Gender Identity (SOGI). The addition of SOGI elements reflected federal civil rights priorities and requires systems to capture both sexual orientation and gender identity as discrete, coded fields separate from sex assigned at birth.

USCDI v3, finalized in July 2022, added eight additional data classes including Facility Information, Specimen, Scan Conversion, Communication, Average Blood Pressure, and Substance Use. It also promoted several elements that had been listed as "emerging" in prior versions. Average Blood Pressure as a distinct element — separate from individual blood pressure observations — reflects clinical evidence that averaged readings are more predictive of cardiovascular risk than single measurements. Each USCDI version is backward-compatible: a system supporting v3 must also support all elements from v1 and v2.

ONC's Annual Update Rule links USCDI versioning to the certification criteria for EHR technology. Certified health IT must demonstrate support for the USCDI version in effect at the time of certification. CHDA candidates must know which data classes were introduced at each version, because exam questions frequently ask which elements are required under a specific regulatory version.

.15 US Core Implementation Guide: Must-Support, Conformance Language, and Profiles

The US Core Implementation Guide (IG) is published by HL7 and maps USCDI data elements to specific FHIR R4 resources and profiles. A profile is a set of constraints applied to a base FHIR resource: it may restrict cardinality (making an optional element required), bind a value set to a coded element, or prohibit certain optional fields. The US Core IG is the implementation-level bridge between USCDI policy requirements and FHIR technical practice.

Conformance language in US Core follows RFC 2119 keywords with precise meanings. SHALL indicates an absolute requirement; a system that does not fulfill a SHALL requirement is non-conformant. SHOULD indicates a strong recommendation that may be deviated from with justification. MAY describes optional behavior. These keywords appear in IG narrative and are also encoded in the StructureDefinition resource that formally defines each profile.

The must-support flag (MS) is the most important concept for CHDA candidates to understand. In US Core, a must-support element is one that a sending system SHALL populate if the information is available and a receiving system SHALL be capable of storing and displaying. Critically, must-support does not mean the element is always required to be present; it means both sides of an exchange must be capable of handling it. For example, the US Core Patient profile marks race and ethnicity as must-support. A system that holds race data must include it in transmitted records; a receiving system must be able to accept and display that data. However, a patient record that genuinely lacks a documented race value may omit the element without violating the profile.

US Core defines profiles for all USCDI data classes. The US Core Condition profile requires the clinicalStatus and verificationStatus coded elements (both bound to specific value sets from the FHIR core terminology), a code element bound to SNOMED CT or ICD-10-CM, and subject and encounter references. The US Core MedicationRequest profile requires medication (either a coded reference or a text string), subject, encounter, requester, and authoredOn. The US Core DiagnosticReport profile for laboratory results requires a code, status, subject, effective date, and at least one result reference to an Observation resource.

Terminology binding strength is another conformance concept tested on the exam. A required binding means the coded value must come from the specified value set, with no exceptions. An extensible binding means the code must come from the value set if an applicable code exists; if none fits, a local code may be used. A preferred binding is a recommendation without enforcement. A example binding provides a sample value set for guidance only.

Exam Tip: Know that must-support in US Core creates bilateral obligations — both sender and receiver — and does not equate to the element being required in every exchange. Exam distractors often conflate must-support with cardinality of 1..1 (required). Must-support and required cardinality are independent flags.

.16 C-CDA and CDA Documents: CCD, Discharge Summary, and Referral Note

Clinical Document Architecture (CDA) is an HL7 standard (originally HL7 v3) that defines the structure and semantics of clinical documents for exchange. CDA documents are XML files with a hierarchical structure: a header containing metadata (document type, author, custodian, patient identification, effective time) and a body containing one or more sections, each identified by an LOINC code. Consolidated CDA (C-CDA) is an HL7 implementation guide published by ONC that standardizes the templates — specific structural patterns — for the most common clinical document types used in the United States.

C-CDA 2.1 is the version referenced by ONC certification criteria. It defines templates at the document, section, and entry level. Document templates specify which sections are required, which are optional, and which are prohibited. Section templates specify how data within each section must be structured. Entry templates define machine-readable representations of discrete clinical data within a narrative section. The combination of narrative text and machine-readable entries is what distinguishes C-CDA from plain text documents and enables structured data extraction.

The Continuity of Care Document (CCD) is the most widely used C-CDA document type. Its LOINC code is 34133-9 (Summarization of Episode Note). The CCD is designed for longitudinal patient summary — it contains a snapshot of the patient's health status spanning all time, not a single encounter. Required sections include Allergies and Intolerances, Medications, Problems, and Results. Optional sections include Procedures, Immunizations, Vital Signs, and Social History. The CCD is the document type used for transitions of care as required under Meaningful Use and the Cures Rule, and it is what a patient receives when requesting their full health record summary.

The Discharge Summary (LOINC 18842-5) is triggered by inpatient hospital discharge. It must capture the reason for admission, hospital course, significant findings, discharge diagnosis, discharge condition, discharge instructions, attending physician, discharge medications, and follow-up plan. Unlike the CCD, the Discharge Summary is encounter-specific and describes what happened during the hospitalization.

The Referral Note (LOINC 57133-1) is triggered when a provider refers a patient to another provider or specialist for evaluation or treatment. It contains the reason for referral, relevant medical history, current medications, allergies, and the specific question the referring provider wants the specialist to address. The Referral Note travels from the referring provider to the receiving provider at the point of referral, before the specialist encounter occurs.

A fourth document type frequently tested is the Progress Note (LOINC 11506-3), which documents a single outpatient encounter or inpatient daily assessment. Knowing the LOINC code and clinical trigger for each document type is essential exam preparation.

.17 Direct Messaging, Care Transitions, TEFCA, and QHIN Enrollment

Direct messaging — formally called the Direct Project — is a federally specified protocol for point-to-point secure messaging between healthcare entities. It operates over SMTP (Simple Mail Transfer Protocol) with S/MIME (Secure/Multipurpose Internet Mail Extensions) encryption layered on top. Each participant in the Direct network holds a Direct address (formatted like an email address, e.g., provider@direct.hospital.org) and an X.509 digital certificate issued by a trusted certificate authority. When a sender transmits a Direct message, the message is encrypted with the recipient's public key and signed with the sender's private key, ensuring both confidentiality and sender authentication.

Direct messaging is the transmission protocol specified by ONC for Transitions of Care under the Meaningful Use (and subsequently Promoting Interoperability) programs. A Transition of Care is defined as the movement of a patient from one care setting to another: hospital to primary care, primary care to specialist, acute care to skilled nursing facility. Under Stage 2 Meaningful Use, eligible hospitals were required to electronically transmit a C-CDA (typically a CCD or Discharge Summary) using Direct for a specified percentage of transitions. The C-CDA document carries the clinical content; Direct is the secure transmission envelope.

Health Information Service Providers (HISPs) are organizations that operate Direct messaging infrastructure — managing certificate issuance, message routing, and security on behalf of providers. Providers typically contract with a HISP rather than operating their own Direct infrastructure.

The Trusted Exchange Framework and Common Agreement (TEFCA) is ONC's framework, published under the 21st Century Cures Act, for creating a universal floor for nationwide health information exchange. TEFCA operates through Qualified Health Information Networks (QHINs) — nationally scaled networks that sign a Common Agreement with ONC's designated coordinating entity (The Sequoia Project). As of 2026, enrolled QHINs include eHealth Exchange, Epic's Carequality-aligned network, CommonWell Health Alliance, Kno2, MedAllies, and Health Gorilla, among others.

Under TEFCA, a covered entity or their designated network connects to a QHIN, which then enables exchange with all other QHINs and their participants through a single on-ramp. TEFCA defines five exchange purposes: Treatment, Individual Access Services (patient-mediated), Payment and Healthcare Operations, Public Health, and Government Benefits Determination. Each purpose carries specific permitted uses and limitations.

QHIN enrollment requires execution of the TEFCA Common Agreement, technical onboarding to the QHIN's infrastructure, and compliance with the Qualified Health Information Network Technical Framework (QTF), which specifies minimum technical, security, and operational requirements including FHIR APIs, audit logging, and patient matching.

.18 ONC Cures Rule API Requirements: Patient, Provider, and Payer-to-Payer Exchange

The ONC 21st Century Cures Act Final Rule (85 FR 25642), effective April 2021 for most provisions, established three distinct API mandates tied to certified health IT and, separately, to payers regulated under CMS. Understanding which mandate applies to which entity and what it requires is critical for the CHDA exam.

The Patient Access API is required for both certified health IT (under ONC) and for payers (under the CMS Interoperability and Patient Access Rule). Certified EHR technology must provide patients with access to their electronic health information through a standardized FHIR R4 API without special effort. This means the EHR must expose a patient-facing FHIR endpoint secured with SMART on FHIR, allowing patients to authorize third-party applications to retrieve their data. The patient's right to this access derives from the HIPAA Right of Access and is reinforced by the Cures Rule's information blocking prohibition.

For payers regulated under the CMS Interoperability Rule (CMS-9115-F, applicable to Medicare Advantage, Medicaid managed care, CHIP, and Qualified Health Plans on Federally Facilitated Exchanges), the Patient Access API must expose claims and encounter data, formulary data, and clinical data (where available) through a FHIR R4 API. Members must be able to authorize third-party apps to retrieve their data. Payers were required to implement their Patient Access API by January 1, 2021.

The Provider Access API, required under CMS rulemaking effective January 1, 2027 for most payers, requires payers to share patient data with treating providers upon request. When a provider queries the payer's FHIR endpoint with the patient's consent, the payer must return claims, encounter, and clinical data relevant to care coordination. This API is bidirectional in concept: it enables providers to receive payer-held information that may not be present in their own EHR, such as out-of-network encounters.

Payer-to-Payer Exchange requires payers to share patient data when a patient changes health plans. When a patient enrolls in a new plan and requests that their historical data be transferred, the old payer must transmit up to five years of claims and clinical data to the new payer within one business day. The technical mechanism is a FHIR API exchange, and the content must include at minimum the data classes in USCDI v1. This requirement addresses the long-standing gap in which patients who changed insurers lost access to historical claims and care context.

The Information Blocking Rule, finalized concurrently, prohibits healthcare providers, health IT developers, and health information networks from engaging in practices that interfere with the access, exchange, or use of electronic health information unless the practice falls within one of eight statutory exceptions (including preventing harm, privacy, security, infeasibility, health IT performance, content and manner, fees, and licensing). Violations are subject to civil monetary penalties enforced by the Office of Inspector General (OIG) for providers and the Office of the National Coordinator for certified health IT developers.

Exam Tip: The CHDA exam tests the distinction between the ONC Cures Rule (which governs certified health IT developers and health information networks) and the CMS Interoperability Rule (which governs payers). Both rules reference FHIR R4 APIs and USCDI, but their enforcement mechanisms and covered entities differ. Providers are subject to the information blocking prohibition but are not required to implement APIs themselves — their EHR vendors are.

.19 Key Concepts

- FHIR resources are modular, web-native clinical data units; R4 is the ONC-mandated version; R5 is current but not yet federally required for API compliance.
- SMART on FHIR scopes follow the pattern patient/[ResourceType].[read|write|*]; the EHR launch context passes a launch token to convey current patient and encounter without user prompting.
- USCDI v1 established 12 data classes; v2 added SOGI, pediatric vital signs, and encounter information; v3 added average blood pressure and substance use — each version is backward-compatible with all prior versions.
- US Core must-support creates bilateral obligations on sender and receiver but does not require the element to be present in every instance; it is independent of element cardinality.
- C-CDA document type selection is driven by the clinical trigger event: CCD (34133-9) for longitudinal summary, Discharge Summary (18842-5) for hospital discharge, Referral Note (57133-1) for specialist referral.
- Direct messaging uses SMTP + S/MIME with X.509 certificates; HISPs manage infrastructure and certificate issuance on behalf of provider organizations.
- TEFCA QHINs provide a single on-ramp to nationwide exchange under a Common Agreement; enrolled QHINs as of 2026 include eHealth Exchange, Epic, CommonWell, and others.
- The ONC Cures Rule's information blocking prohibition covers providers, health IT developers, and health information networks, with eight statutory exceptions; enforcement of provider violations rests with OIG.

.20 Chapter 9 Review Questions

1. A hospital EHR vendor publishes a FHIR R4 endpoint. A developer queries the URL /Patient/12345 using an HTTP GET. Which FHIR interaction type does this represent?

A. Search
B. Read
C. Create
D. Retrieve-all

Correct answer: B. A GET request to a resource type followed by a logical ID (e.g., /Patient/12345) is the FHIR READ interaction, which returns a single resource by its server-assigned identifier. The SEARCH interaction uses GET with query parameters (e.g., /Patient?family=Smith) and returns a Bundle. CREATE uses HTTP POST. "Retrieve-all" is not a defined FHIR interaction.

2. Under USCDI v2, which data class was added that was NOT present in USCDI v1?

A. Vital Signs
B. Medications
C. Sexual Orientation and Gender Identity
D. Allergies and Intolerances

Correct answer: C. Sexual Orientation and Gender Identity (SOGI) was introduced as a new data class in USCDI v2 (July 2021). Vital Signs, Medications, and Allergies and Intolerances were all present in USCDI v1. CHDA candidates must distinguish which data classes belong to each version because exam questions frequently use version-specific membership as a testable point.

3. A care coordinator receives a C-CDA document following a patient's inpatient hospital stay. The document contains reason for admission, hospital course, and discharge medications. Which document type is this?

A. Continuity of Care Document
B. Referral Note
C. Discharge Summary
D. Progress Note

Correct answer: C. The Discharge Summary (LOINC 18842-5) is the C-CDA document type triggered by inpatient hospital discharge and must include reason for admission, hospital course, discharge diagnosis, and discharge medications. The CCD (34133-9) is a longitudinal patient summary not tied to a single encounter. The Referral Note is sent before a specialist encounter, not after hospitalization. The Progress Note documents a single outpatient or inpatient daily assessment.

4. In the US Core Implementation Guide, a data element flagged as must-support requires which of the following?

A. The element must be present with a non-null value in every transmitted resource instance.
B. Both sending and receiving systems must be capable of handling the element.
C. The element must be bound to a required terminology value set.
D. The element cardinality must be set to 1..1 in the profile.

Correct answer: B. Must-support in US Core creates bilateral obligations: a sender must populate the element when the information is available, and a receiver must be capable of storing and rendering it. Must-support does not require the element to appear in every instance (that is determined by cardinality), does not mandate a specific terminology binding, and does not fix cardinality at 1..1. These are independent profile constraints.

5. A provider wants to send a patient's clinical summary to a specialist using Direct messaging. Which encryption and signature standard does Direct messaging use?

A. TLS with RSA-2048 at the connection layer only
B. PGP (Pretty Good Privacy) with shared symmetric keys
C. S/MIME with X.509 digital certificates
D. OAuth 2.0 bearer tokens over HTTPS

Correct answer: C. Direct messaging uses SMTP as the transport protocol with S/MIME (Secure/Multipurpose Internet Mail Extensions) for end-to-end encryption and digital signatures, relying on X.509 certificates issued by trust-anchored certificate authorities. TLS provides transport-layer security for many protocols but is not the application-layer security mechanism specified by Direct. PGP is not part of the Direct specification. OAuth 2.0 is an authorization framework used with FHIR APIs, not Direct messaging.

6. Under the ONC 21st Century Cures Act Final Rule, which entity is primarily responsible for providing a patient-facing FHIR R4 API that allows third-party application access?

A. The covered provider organization
B. The certified health IT developer
C. The state health information exchange
D. The QHIN serving the provider

Correct answer: B. The ONC Cures Rule places the obligation to implement and maintain the patient-facing FHIR R4 API on certified health IT developers (EHR vendors), not on the provider organizations that use their software. Providers are subject to the information blocking prohibition but are not independently required to build or host APIs. State HIEs and QHINs serve exchange functions but are not the regulated entity for this specific API requirement.

7. Which TEFCA exchange purpose permits a health information network to share patient data with a public health agency for disease surveillance without patient authorization?

A. Individual Access Services
B. Treatment
C. Public Health
D. Government Benefits Determination

Correct answer: C. TEFCA defines Public Health as one of five permitted exchange purposes, allowing QHINs and their participants to share patient data with authorized public health entities for surveillance, reporting, and response activities without individual patient authorization, consistent with HIPAA public health activity permissions. Individual Access Services is patient-mediated access. Treatment requires a provider relationship. Government Benefits Determination applies to eligibility and enrollment for programs such as Medicaid.

8. A FHIR server's CapabilityStatement lists a binding strength of "extensible" for the Condition.code element. What does this mean for a sending system?

A. The code must always come from the specified value set with no exceptions.
B. A code from the value set must be used if one applies; a local code is permissible if no applicable code exists.
C. The code should come from the value set as a recommendation, but local codes are freely permitted.
D. Any code from any code system is acceptable; the value set is provided as an example only.

Correct answer: B. An extensible binding requires use of a value set code when a clinically appropriate code exists within the value set. If the concept genuinely cannot be represented by any value set member, a local or alternative code is permissible. Required binding allows no exceptions. Preferred binding is a recommendation without enforcement. Example binding provides the value set for illustrative purposes only and imposes no obligation.

9. Under the CMS Interoperability and Patient Access Rule, which data elements must a regulated payer expose through its Patient Access API at minimum?

A. Claims and encounter data only
B. Claims, encounter data, formulary information, and clinical data where available
C. Clinical data from hospital admissions only, formatted as a Discharge Summary
D. Enrollment and eligibility data only, per the HIPAA transactions standards

Correct answer: B. The CMS Interoperability and Patient Access Rule requires regulated payers (Medicare Advantage, Medicaid managed care, CHIP, and QHP issuers on Federally Facilitated Exchanges) to expose claims and encounter data, formulary data, and clinical data (where available) through a FHIR R4 Patient Access API. The requirement is broader than claims alone and includes formulary information, which is essential for medication management and care transitions. Enrollment data alone would not meet the rule's minimum content requirements.

10. A patient changes health insurance plans. Under the CMS Payer-to-Payer Exchange requirement, what must the previous payer do?

A. Mail a paper summary of the patient's benefits history within 30 days.
B. Share the patient's data with the new payer within one business day of a valid patient request, covering up to five years of claims and clinical data.
C. Notify the patient's providers and wait for provider authorization before releasing data.
D. Transfer data only if the patient submits a written HIPAA authorization to both payers.

Correct answer: B. The CMS Payer-to-Payer Exchange requirement obligates the previous payer to transmit up to five years of the patient's claims and clinical data to the new payer within one business day of a valid patient-initiated request, using a FHIR API. The patient's request serves as the authorization mechanism under the rule; a separate written HIPAA authorization or provider sign-off is not required. The exchange is electronic, not paper-based, and the content must include at minimum USCDI v1 data classes.

Healthcare Data Warehousing and Population Analytics

.21 Learning Objectives

- Distinguish among enterprise data warehouses, data marts, and data lakes in the healthcare context, and explain the role of star and snowflake schemas in dimensional modeling.
- Describe the ETL/ELT pipeline lifecycle—extraction, transformation, loading, and lineage documentation—as applied to EHR, claims, laboratory, and pharmacy source systems.
- Apply risk stratification frameworks (ACG, HCC, and LACE) and attribution methodologies to identify high-risk patients and care gaps within attributed populations.
- Explain how social determinants of health are captured through ICD-10-CM Z codes, PRAPARE, and AHC HRSN screening instruments, and integrated into population analytics.
- Design population health dashboards that incorporate HEDIS measures, benchmark comparisons, and stratification by race/ethnicity and payer in alignment with equity and value-based care requirements.

.22 Data Warehouse Architecture in Healthcare

A healthcare data warehouse is a subject-oriented, integrated, nonvolatile, and time-variant repository that consolidates clinical, administrative, and financial data to support analytical decision-making. Understanding its architectural forms is fundamental to the CHDA examination.

Dimensional Modeling Fundamentals. The most widely used approach to organizing analytical data is dimensional modeling, developed by Ralph Kimball. The two core schemas are the star schema and the snowflake schema. In a star schema, a central fact table—containing measurable events such as hospitalizations, lab results, or claims payments—connects directly to surrounding dimension tables that describe context: patient demographics, provider attributes, time periods, and diagnosis codes. The design is denormalized for query speed. In a snowflake schema, dimension tables are further normalized into sub-dimensions; for instance, a Diagnosis dimension might link to a separate ICD-10 hierarchy table. The snowflake reduces data redundancy but requires more complex joins. In healthcare, star schemas dominate analytics environments because query performance is paramount and storage costs are relatively low.

Enterprise Data Warehouse vs. Data Mart vs. Data Lake. These three structures serve distinct purposes and are often deployed together. An enterprise data warehouse (EDW) is an organization-wide, historically complete repository integrating data from all operational source systems—EHRs, practice management systems, lab information systems, and claims processors. It enforces enterprise-wide data governance standards and serves as the single version of truth for reporting across departments. A data mart is a subset of the EDW scoped to a specific department, specialty, or analytic domain (e.g., a cardiology quality data mart or a payer-specific cost data mart). Data marts accelerate departmental reporting by pre-aggregating commonly used measures and limiting access to relevant data elements. A data lake is a scalable storage environment—often cloud-based—that ingests raw, unstructured, and semi-structured data at low cost without requiring upfront schema definition. Healthcare organizations use data lakes to store unprocessed FHIR bundles, genomic files, imaging metadata, and wearable device streams. The lake feeds transformation pipelines that ultimately load structured analytic tables into the EDW.

Temporal Design. Healthcare warehouses require robust handling of slowly changing dimensions—for example, a patient's insurance coverage or primary care attribution that changes over time. Slowly Changing Dimension Type 2 (SCD2) is the standard approach: when a dimension attribute changes, a new row is inserted with updated effective and expiration date columns, preserving the full history. This is essential for accurate retrospective quality measurement.

Exam Tip: On CHDA exam questions contrasting EDW, data mart, and data lake, remember that only the EDW enforces enterprise-wide governance and integration. Data lakes store raw data without schema enforcement; data marts serve departmental subsets with pre-aggregated measures.

.23 ETL/ELT Processes in Healthcare Analytics

Moving data from operational source systems into an analytical repository involves extraction, transformation, and loading (ETL) or, in modern cloud architectures, extraction, loading, and then transformation (ELT). The order matters because ELT leverages the processing power of cloud data platforms to transform data after it has landed in the target environment.

Extraction. Healthcare source systems include EHRs (Epic, Oracle Health/Cerner, Meditech), claims processing systems (payer adjudication platforms), laboratory information systems (LIS), pharmacy dispensing systems, and registration/scheduling modules. Extraction methods vary by source: HL7 v2 message feeds deliver ADT (Admit-Discharge-Transfer) and ORU (observation result) messages in near real time; FHIR APIs enable structured RESTful queries against operational data; flat-file extracts (CSV, pipe-delimited) are common for claims and pharmacy; database replication captures changes via transaction logs (CDC, or change data capture). Clinical data analysts must understand that extraction scope is governed by data use agreements, particularly when claims data is received from health plans or CMS.

Transformation. Raw source data is rarely analytics-ready. Transformation rules address: standardizing date formats, normalizing code systems (mapping local charge codes to CPT, SNOMED CT, or LOINC), deduplicating patient records through probabilistic or deterministic matching using master patient index (MPI) algorithms, applying business logic (e.g., defining a "readmission" as an inpatient admission within 30 days of discharge for the same or related condition), and deriving calculated fields (length of stay, total cost of care). Transformation logic must be documented formally because regulators and accrediting bodies require auditability.

Load Schedules. Incremental loads (delta loads) append only newly created or modified records since the last extraction. Full refreshes replace the target table entirely and are used for small dimension tables or when source systems cannot provide reliable change indicators. Load timing matters: claims data typically arrives with a 30–90 day lag for adjudication, whereas EHR encounter data may be available within 24 hours. Analytics depending on claims for cost attribution must account for claims run-out and incurred-but-not-reported (IBNR) liabilities.

Data Lineage. Lineage documentation traces each data element from its original source system through every transformation step to its final analytic use. Tools such as Apache Atlas, Collibra, or Alation provide automated lineage capture. For the CHDA, lineage supports three governance requirements: data quality auditing, regulatory compliance (particularly for HIPAA minimum necessary), and reproducibility of quality measurement calculations when presented to CMS, accreditors, or legal proceedings.

.24 Population Health Analytics: Risk Stratification and Care Gap Identification

Population health management requires identifying patients who are at elevated risk for high-cost events—hospitalizations, emergency department visits, disease progression—before those events occur. Risk stratification is the analytic foundation for this work.

ACG System. The Johns Hopkins Adjusted Clinical Groups (ACG) system uses ambulatory diagnosis codes to assign patients to morbidity groups based on resource utilization expectations. ACG weights reflect the chronic disease burden and expected cost associated with each group. The system is particularly useful for primary care-based population health programs and for capitation rate setting in value-based contracts.

HCC Model. The CMS Hierarchical Condition Category (HCC) model, used in Medicare Advantage risk adjustment, assigns diagnosis codes to condition categories that are then grouped hierarchically (so that a more severe manifestation supersedes a less severe one). Each HCC carries a relative factor; the sum of a beneficiary's demographic and HCC factors produces a risk adjustment factor (RAF) score that determines capitated payment. Organizations managing Medicare populations must ensure coding completeness—undercoded conditions yield lower RAF scores and inadequate capitation revenue.

LACE Index. The LACE tool is a readmission risk model calculated at discharge using four variables: Length of stay, Acuity of admission (emergency vs. elective), Comorbidity burden (Charlson Comorbidity Index), and Emergency department use in the prior six months. Scores of 10 or higher designate high readmission risk. LACE is actionable at the point of discharge planning, making it a widely deployed tool in care transition programs.

Attribution Methodologies. Attribution assigns patients to a responsible provider or care team for purposes of accountability measurement. Plurality attribution assigns the patient to the provider who delivered the most primary care visits in the measurement period. Sequential attribution first checks for a primary care provider of record, then falls to plurality. CMS uses plurality attribution for ACO quality programs. Attribution methodology directly affects denominator construction in quality measures: the same patient may appear in different providers' panels depending on attribution rules.

Care Gap Identification. A care gap exists when a patient who meets a measure's denominator eligibility has not received the required service. Automated care gap registries query the warehouse nightly, joining patient eligibility, diagnosis history, and service utilization to flag overdue preventive or chronic disease management services—such as HbA1c testing for patients with diabetes, annual retinal exams, or colorectal cancer screening.

.25 Social Determinants of Health Data: Coding, Screening, and Integration

Social determinants of health (SDOH) are the nonmedical conditions in which people are born, grow, live, work, and age. They include housing instability, food insecurity, transportation barriers, interpersonal violence, and social isolation. The healthcare system's ability to address SDOH at scale depends on structured data capture and analytic integration.

Z Codes in ICD-10-CM. ICD-10-CM Chapter 21 (Z00–Z99) includes a dedicated subcategory for SDOH: the Z55–Z65 codes cover education, employment, housing, financial, family, interpersonal, and psychosocial circumstances. For example, Z59.0 designates homelessness, Z59.4 lack of adequate food, and Z63.4 disappearance of family member. CMS encouraged Z code use in the 2019 IPPS rule; CMS-HCC V28 (effective 2024) incorporated select SDOH diagnoses into the risk adjustment model. Despite this encouragement, Z code capture rates remain low in most organizations—studies report capture on fewer than 2% of encounters where a social need is present—because clinical workflows do not reliably prompt documentation.

Screening Tools. Structured screening instruments standardize SDOH data collection at the point of care. PRAPARE (Protocol for Responding to and Assessing Patients' Assets, Risks, and Experiences), developed by the National Association of Community Health Centers, contains 21 items covering national origin, housing, employment, insurance, farm work, and other domains. The AHC HRSN (Accountable Health Communities Health-Related Social Needs) screening tool, developed by CMS, uses 10 core questions to identify needs in five domains: housing, food, transportation, utilities, and interpersonal safety. The AHC tool is required for organizations participating in the CMS Accountable Health Communities Model. Both instruments are mapped to Z codes and LOINC codes to enable structured electronic documentation.

Incorporating SDOH into Analytics. SDOH data can be incorporated at individual and community levels. Individual-level SDOH comes from screening instruments and Z codes. Community-level proxies include census tract-based indices such as the Area Deprivation Index (ADI), the Social Vulnerability Index (SVI), and the Child Opportunity Index (COI). These indices are joined to patient records via geocoded address, allowing analysts to estimate social risk even when individual screening data is absent. Multivariable risk models that incorporate SDOH alongside clinical variables consistently outperform clinical-only models in predicting ED utilization, readmissions, and medication nonadherence. The CHDA must understand that SDOH data integration raises data governance questions: consent for sharing social needs data with community partners, minimum necessary standards under HIPAA, and equity implications of using socioeconomic proxies in clinical risk scores.

Exam Tip: Know that Z codes from ICD-10-CM Chapter 21 are the primary mechanism for documenting individual SDOH in the medical record. PRAPARE and AHC HRSN are the two screening tools most likely to appear on the CHDA exam. The Area Deprivation Index provides community-level SDOH through census-tract geocoding when individual screening data is unavailable.

.26 Clinical and Claims Data Integration

Comprehensive population analytics requires combining clinical data from EHRs with administrative claims data from payers. Each source has strengths and limitations; neither alone provides a complete picture of patient health and utilization.

Clinical Data Characteristics. EHR data captures the richness of the clinical encounter: problem lists, vital signs, laboratory values, medication orders, and free-text notes. Clinical data is often more granular and timely than claims. However, EHR data reflects only the services rendered within a single health system's network.

A patient who receives specialist care at a competing health system or fills prescriptions at an out-of-network pharmacy is invisible in the EHR alone. Clinical data also reflects documentation behavior—ICD-10 codes on problem lists may lag behind the actual encounter notes, and social history fields are notoriously incomplete.

Claims Data Characteristics. Adjudicated claims data, typically received from commercial payers, Medicare, or Medicaid, captures services across all network providers and facilities, making it far superior for total cost of care analysis and out-of-network utilization tracking. Claims are structured (837 institutional and 837 professional formats, or equivalents) and include procedure codes (CPT/HCPCS), diagnosis codes (ICD-10-CM), revenue codes, place of service, and paid amounts. Claims arrive with a lag: professional claims are typically adjudicated in 30–45 days; institutional claims may take 60–90 days. This lag must be accounted for in period-of-analysis definitions.

Pharmacy Data. Pharmacy claims (NCPDP format) provide medication dispensing records including NDC code, days supply, quantity dispensed, and prescribing provider. Medication adherence measures—such as Proportion of Days Covered (PDC)—are calculated exclusively from pharmacy claims, not from EHR prescribing data. PDC is the standard measure used in HEDIS for statin therapy, RAAS antagonists, and diabetes medications.

Attributed Population Construction. Building an attributed population for an ACO, value-based contract, or quality reporting program requires: defining the eligibility window (e.g., continuously enrolled for 11 of 12 months), applying attribution logic (plurality, sequential, or voluntary attestation), excluding members with Medicare Part A and Part B in parallel if the contract is MSSP, and linking clinical and claims records using enterprise master patient index (EMPI) matching. The result is a denominator-ready population file that feeds downstream measure calculations and risk stratification algorithms.

.27 Dashboard Design for Population Health

Population health dashboards translate complex analytics into actionable operational intelligence for clinical leaders, care managers, and executives. Effective dashboard design follows principles of measure selection, visual hierarchy, and equity-focused stratification.

Measure Selection. Dashboards should display measures that are actionable, evidence-based, and aligned with contractual or regulatory obligations. HEDIS (Healthcare Effectiveness Data and Information Set) measures, maintained by NCQA, are the most widely used standardized quality measures in U.S. healthcare and cover domains including preventive care, chronic disease management, behavioral health access, and patient experience. Examples include Controlling High Blood Pressure (CBP), Diabetes Care—HbA1c Poor Control (HBD), and Antidepressant Medication Management (AMM). HEDIS technical specifications govern numerator and denominator definitions precisely, and the CHDA must follow them to produce auditable rates. Beyond HEDIS, dashboards may include CMS Star Ratings measures for Medicare Advantage, Core Set measures for Medicaid, and internally defined operational metrics such as care management outreach completion rates.

Benchmark Comparison. Measures displayed without context are difficult to interpret. Dashboards should include benchmark comparisons at minimum three levels: the organization's own prior-period performance (trend line), regional or state-level averages from AHRQ or state health data organizations, and national HEDIS percentile benchmarks published annually by NCQA (25th, 50th, 75th, and 90th percentiles by product line). Displaying current performance against the NCQA 75th percentile target motivates improvement teams and supports strategic goal setting.

Stratification by Race/Ethnicity and Payer. Aggregate quality rates mask disparities. Dashboard stratification by race/ethnicity, language preference, payer/product line, and geography (census tract or ZIP code) is now an expectation under CMS health equity frameworks and NCQA HEDIS Disparities Reporting. The CMS Race and Ethnicity Data Disparities Improvement methodology uses an enhanced algorithm to impute race/ethnicity for Medicare beneficiaries using name and geography when self-reported data is missing. Organizations must also comply with the updated UDS+ data standards and the CMS disparities roadmap, which require disaggregated reporting at granular race/ethnicity categories rather than aggregated OMB categories.

Exam Tip: HEDIS measures are the most exam-relevant quality framework for population health dashboards. Know that PDC is the standard adherence measure for medications, that NCQA publishes national benchmarks at the 25th/50th/75th/90th percentiles, and that equity stratification by race/ethnicity is now a regulatory expectation rather than optional best practice.

Interactivity and Usability. Effective dashboards use drill-down capability so that a care manager can move from a population-level CBP rate to a list of patients whose most recent blood pressure reading exceeds 140/90.

Color conventions should be consistent and accessibility-aware (colorblind-safe palettes). Alert thresholds should trigger proactive notifications when a measure crosses below a predefined floor. Dashboard governance—defining ownership, update frequency, and version control for measure logic—prevents the proliferation of conflicting numbers across the organization.

.28 Key Concepts

- **Star schema**: Dimensional model with a central fact table joined directly to denormalized dimension tables; optimized for query speed in analytical environments.
- **Snowflake schema**: Normalized variant of the star schema in which dimension tables are further decomposed into sub-dimensions; reduces redundancy but increases join complexity.
- **ETL vs. ELT**: ETL transforms data before loading (traditional on-premise warehouses); ELT loads raw data first and transforms within the target platform (modern cloud architectures).
- **HCC risk adjustment**: CMS model using hierarchical condition categories derived from ICD-10-CM diagnoses to calculate a risk adjustment factor (RAF) score for Medicare Advantage capitation.
- **LACE Index**: Discharge readmission risk tool scored on Length of stay, Acuity, Comorbidity (Charlson), and Emergency department use; scores ≥10 indicate high risk.
- **Z codes (ICD-10-CM Z55–Z65)**: The primary structured mechanism for documenting social determinants of health in the medical record, including housing, food, employment, and interpersonal circumstances.
- **Proportion of Days Covered (PDC)**: Pharmacy claims–based adherence metric; the standard measure for HEDIS medication management domains including statins, RAAS antagonists, and diabetes medications.
- **Care gap registry**: A query-driven list of patients who meet a quality measure denominator but have not yet received the required service; used operationally by care management teams to drive outreach.

.29 Chapter 10 Review Questions

1. A health system is designing an analytical repository that must serve both enterprise-wide reporting and department-specific dashboards for cardiology and oncology. Which architecture best supports both requirements?

A. A single data lake with no schema enforcement
B. An enterprise data warehouse with department-specific data marts
C. Separate operational databases for each department
D. A snowflake schema database with no upstream EDW

Correct Answer: B. An EDW provides the integrated, governed, enterprise-wide repository that enforces a single version of truth across all departments. Department-specific data marts are built on top of the EDW, providing pre-aggregated, scoped datasets that accelerate cardiology and oncology reporting. A data lake (A) is appropriate for raw, unstructured data storage but cannot serve as the governed analytic layer. Separate operational databases (C) create silos and prevent enterprise integration. A standalone snowflake schema (D) addresses only dimensional modeling design, not the governance and integration requirements described.

2. An ACO is calculating a Medicare beneficiary's capitation payment under the CMS Medicare Advantage model. The patient has diagnoses of Type 2 diabetes with diabetic chronic kidney disease (E11.22) and hypertension (I10). Under the HCC model, how are these conditions handled?

A. Each diagnosis contributes an independent additive HCC factor
B. The hierarchical structure selects only the most severe condition within each category, suppressing lesser diagnoses
C. Only diagnoses documented in the current year's inpatient claims are eligible
D. Hypertension is excluded from HCC scoring because it is too prevalent

Correct Answer: B. The HCC model is hierarchical: within a disease group, only the most severe condition category is counted, preventing double-counting. E11.22 maps to a more specific diabetic CKD HCC that subsumes the general diabetes HCC. The two conditions (diabetes/CKD and hypertension) are in different disease groups and both contribute factors, but within any single group the hierarchy applies. Answer A incorrectly suggests all diagnoses add independently with no suppression. Answer C is incorrect; HCC uses any Part A or B claim, professional claim, or encounter data. Answer D is incorrect; hypertension is an eligible HCC diagnosis.

3. A clinical informatics analyst is building a data pipeline from a hospital EHR. The source system provides HL7 v2 ADT messages for patient movements and flat-file lab extracts. The analyst needs to document each data element's path from source to final analytic table. What governance artifact does this produce?

A. Data dictionary
B. Entity-relationship diagram
C. Data lineage map
D. Master patient index

Correct Answer: C. Data lineage documentation traces each field from its origin (e.g., HL7 v2 ADT PID segment for patient demographics) through every transformation step to its final destination in the analytics warehouse. Lineage supports auditability, regulatory compliance, and reproducibility of quality measure calculations. A data dictionary (A) defines field meanings, types, and allowable values but does not trace transformation flow. An entity-relationship diagram (B) models database relationships. An MPI (D) is used for patient identity matching, not transformation tracing.

4. A care manager receives a care gap report showing that a 58-year-old patient with Type 2 diabetes has not had an HbA1c test in 14 months. The patient is attributed to the practice under a plurality attribution rule. Which of the following best describes the basis for this attribution?

A. The patient designated this practice as their primary care provider in a written attestation
B. The practice billed the highest number of primary care evaluation and management visits for this patient in the measurement period
C. The practice is the nearest geographically to the patient's home address
D. The patient had at least one inpatient admission at the affiliated hospital

Correct Answer: B. Plurality attribution assigns patients to the provider who furnished the greatest number of qualifying primary care visits (typically E&M codes billed by primary care specialties) during the measurement period—regardless of any patient designation. Voluntary attestation (A) describes a different, less common attribution method used in some ACO contracts. Geographic proximity (C) is not an attribution method in standard CMS programs. Inpatient admissions (D) are not a basis for primary care attribution.

5. During a population health data integration project, the analytics team receives adjudicated commercial claims from three payers. The data must be linked to EHR records for the same patients. What is the primary technical mechanism used to match records across these disparate sources?

A. Health plan member ID
B. Social Security Number
C. Enterprise Master Patient Index (EMPI) probabilistic matching
D. National Provider Identifier (NPI)

Correct Answer: C. An EMPI uses probabilistic or deterministic algorithms—comparing name, date of birth, gender, address, and other identifiers—to create a unique enterprise patient identifier that links records across EHRs, claims, and other source systems. Health plan member IDs (A) are payer-specific and do not link across EHRs or different payers. SSN (B) is rarely transmitted in claims and is a high-sensitivity PII element that organizations avoid using as a matching key. NPI (D) identifies providers, not patients.

6. A population health analyst is asked to calculate medication adherence for patients with diabetes on metformin. Which data source is required, and which metric is standard?

A. EHR medication order data; Medication Possession Ratio (MPR)
B. Pharmacy claims (NCPDP); Proportion of Days Covered (PDC)
C. EHR problem list diagnoses; Charlson Comorbidity Index
D. Adjudicated medical claims (837P); Days Supply calculation

Correct Answer: B. HEDIS and virtually all value-based contract adherence measures use PDC calculated from pharmacy dispensing claims in NCPDP format. PDC measures the proportion of days in the measurement period for which the patient had medication on hand, based on fill dates and days supply. EHR medication orders (A) reflect prescribing intent, not actual dispensing, and are not the standard for adherence measurement. Charlson (C) is a comorbidity scoring tool, not an adherence metric. Medical claims (D) do not contain pharmacy dispensing data.

7. An organization is incorporating SDOH data into a risk stratification model for Medicaid patients. Individual-level SDOH screening data is available for only 40% of the population. What approach allows the remaining 60% to receive a community-level SDOH score?

A. Impute missing Z codes from diagnosis history
B. Assign all unscreened patients to the lowest-risk SDOH category

C. Geocode patient addresses and join to the Area Deprivation Index (ADI) by census tract
D. Exclude unscreened patients from SDOH-enhanced models

Correct Answer: C. The Area Deprivation Index, derived from census data, provides a validated community-level measure of socioeconomic disadvantage linked to census tract via geocoded address. This is the standard methodology for imputing SDOH when individual screening data is absent. Imputing Z codes from diagnosis history (A) would fabricate individual-level SDOH data that was never documented. Assigning all unscreened patients to the lowest risk category (B) would introduce systematic bias against high-need patients who were never screened. Exclusion (D) would reduce model performance and may introduce selection bias.

8. A quality analyst building a population health dashboard wants to show whether the organization's performance on the HEDIS Controlling High Blood Pressure (CBP) measure is above or below national norms. Which benchmarking source provides standardized national percentile comparisons for HEDIS measures?

A. CMS Quality Payment Program (QPP) performance data
B. NCQA's annual HEDIS Quality Compass report
C. AHRQ National Healthcare Quality and Disparities Report
D. The Joint Commission ORYX measure benchmarks

Correct Answer: B. NCQA publishes Quality Compass annually, providing national and regional HEDIS performance distributions—including 25th, 50th, 75th, and 90th percentiles—by product line (HMO, PPO, Medicaid, Medicare). This is the authoritative benchmarking source for HEDIS measures. QPP (A) covers Merit-based Incentive Payment System and Alternative Payment Model data, not HEDIS benchmarks. AHRQ (C) publishes national quality and disparities trend data but not HEDIS-specific percentile benchmarks. ORYX (D) is The Joint Commission's hospital performance measurement system, unrelated to HEDIS.

9. An analyst is reviewing the LACE score for a patient discharged after a five-day inpatient admission for acute exacerbation of heart failure. The admission was through the emergency department, the patient has a Charlson Comorbidity Index of 6, and had three ED visits in the prior six months. What is the correct interpretation of a LACE score of 13?

A. The patient is at low readmission risk and can be discharged with standard follow-up
B. The patient is at high readmission risk and should be referred to a transitional care program
C. The LACE score is invalid because it applies only to elective admissions
D. The score is insufficient to act on without adding HCC risk adjustment

Correct Answer: B. A LACE score of 10 or higher designates high readmission risk. A score of 13 reflects: L=3 (5-day LOS), A=3 (emergency admission), C=5 (CCI of 6), E=2 (3 prior ED visits)—placing this patient firmly in the high-risk category warranting proactive transitional care. Answer A is incorrect; scores ≥10 are high risk. Answer C is incorrect; LACE applies to all acute inpatient admissions, not only elective ones. Answer D is incorrect; LACE is a validated standalone readmission predictor and does not require supplementation with HCC scoring at the point of discharge.

10. A health plan is required under a CMS contract to stratify HEDIS quality measure performance by race and ethnicity, but self-reported race/ethnicity data is missing for 35% of Medicare beneficiaries in the denominator. Which methodology does CMS recommend to address this gap?

A. Exclude members with missing race/ethnicity from stratified reporting
B. Assign all members with missing data to an "Unknown" category and report it separately
C. Use the CMS Race and Ethnicity Data Disparities Improvement algorithm, which imputes race/ethnicity using surname and geography
D. Substitute payer-reported plan enrollment race codes, which are always complete

Correct Answer: C. CMS developed the Race and Ethnicity Data Disparities Improvement (REDI) methodology, which uses a Bayesian indirect estimation approach (a form of BISG—Bayesian Improved Surname Geocoding) to impute race/ethnicity for Medicare beneficiaries lacking self-reported data. This is the required approach under CMS health equity measurement programs. Exclusion (A) would undermine the purpose of disparities reporting and bias results toward more data-complete subgroups. Reporting as "Unknown" (B) does not produce actionable stratified rates. Plan enrollment race codes (D) are often incomplete or inaccurate and are not a substitute for the REDI methodology.

Professional Practice, Ethics, and Career Development in Health Analytics

Exam weight: approximately 8 percent

.30 Learning Objectives

After completing this chapter, you will be able to:

- Apply the seven principles of the AHIMA Code of Ethics to real-world data analyst dilemmas involving unauthorized disclosure, data falsification, and conflicts of interest.
- Describe the CHDA recertification cycle, the required continuing education hours, and the categories of CE that AHIMA accepts.
- Apply the CRISP-DM project management framework to a healthcare analytics project, including project scoping and stakeholder communication practices.
- Select appropriate methods for communicating analytical findings to non-technical executives, including dashboards, narrative summaries, and data storytelling principles.
- Identify emerging leadership roles for health data analysts, relevant professional organizations, and credentials that complement the CHDA.

.31 The AHIMA Code of Ethics: Principles and Analyst Dilemmas

AHIMA adopted its Code of Ethics to establish the professional and ethical expectations for all members and credentialed practitioners regardless of role. For the health data analyst, the Code is not an abstract statement of values — it is an operational guide for navigating decisions that arise in daily practice. The exam tests whether candidates can identify the applicable principle and the correct course of action when presented with a scenario.

The Code rests on seven principles. The first principle requires that members advocate for patients and their rights and interests. For the analyst, this manifests most directly in decisions about secondary use of patient data: a request to use a clinical dataset for a commercial purpose that benefits the organization but offers no clear patient benefit may conflict with this principle even if it satisfies HIPAA's minimum necessary standard.

The second principle states that members put service and health above self-interest. In analytics practice, this becomes concrete when a manager pressures an analyst to adjust a measure — for example, to exclude a subpopulation from a readmission rate calculation because the inclusion would produce an unfavorable result that reflects badly on a service line. The analyst's obligation under the second principle is to resist the pressure and surface the concern through appropriate escalation channels.

The third principle calls for accuracy and truth-telling in professional work. Data falsification — altering a dataset to produce a desired result, excluding inconvenient outliers without documented methodological justification, or misrepresenting the confidence interval of a model's output — is a direct violation. The CHDA exam regularly presents scenarios in which an analyst is asked to make results "look better." The correct response is always refusal and escalation, not compliance.

The fourth principle addresses confidentiality. Unauthorized release of protected health information — sharing a patient-level dataset with a vendor who lacks a business associate agreement, emailing a de-identification failure to an external collaborator, or posting aggregate results in a public presentation when the cell sizes are small enough to enable re-identification — constitutes a breach of confidentiality regardless of intent.

The fifth principle requires that members recognize and manage conflicts of interest. An analyst who has a financial stake in a vendor product being evaluated, or who stands to benefit personally from a particular analytic conclusion, must disclose the conflict and, if the conflict is material, recuse from the work. The disclosure obligation extends to relationships that might be perceived as compromising even if they are not actually compromising.

The sixth principle requires continuous professional development. Analysts who allow their skills to atrophy — relying on methods that are outdated, failing to learn new regulatory requirements, or avoiding engagement with the research literature — are not fulfilling their professional obligations. This principle is the ethical foundation for the CE requirements built into CHDA recertification.

The seventh principle requires that members advance and promote the profession. This includes mentoring, contributing to professional organizations, supporting students, and advocating for the role of health data management in quality and safety.

When a question presents an ethical dilemma, candidates should identify the relevant principle first, then identify which response upholds it. In most scenarios, the correct answer involves disclosure, escalation, or refusal — not compliance with an improper request and not unilateral resolution without documentation.

Exam Tip: When a CHDA question describes a supervisor pressuring an analyst to alter or omit data, the correct answer always involves refusal and escalation through documented channels — not compliance, not resignation, and not silent non-compliance.

.32 CHDA Credential Maintenance: CE Requirements and Recertification

The CHDA is a two-year credential. Recertification occurs on a two-year cycle, with the credential expiration date printed on the certificate. Candidates who allow the credential to lapse without completing recertification must retake the examination; there is no grace period for re-examination eligibility. AHIMA does not administer an automatic extension.

To recertify, credential holders must accumulate 30 continuing education hours over each two-year cycle. AHIMA specifies that all 30 hours must fall within approved CE categories, and at least some of those hours must come from activities that are directly relevant to the CHDA domain competencies. As of the 2026 recertification guidelines, AHIMA accepts CE from the following categories:

AHIMA-sponsored education, including the national convention, regional symposia, the AHIMA Foundation webinar series, and the online learning modules available through the AHIMA Learning Management System. Hours from these sources are accepted without limit.

Education provided by AHIMA-approved CE providers, including universities and colleges, hospital continuing education departments, professional associations recognized by AHIMA, and vendors whose programs have received AHIMA CE approval. Candidates must retain documentation — typically a certificate of completion — for all hours claimed.

Academic coursework at accredited institutions. A three-credit-hour college course counts as 45 CE hours, though the total credit from academic coursework is capped under the current guidelines. Candidates should consult the current AHIMA CE brochure for the applicable cap, as AHIMA periodically revises it.

Publication and presentation. Authoring a peer-reviewed article in an AHIMA-recognized journal, presenting at a national or regional conference, or developing an educational program for CE credit earns CE hours. The specific hour equivalents for publication and presentation are detailed in the AHIMA CE brochure.

Volunteer service. Serving on an AHIMA committee, task force, or board of directors earns CE. The hours are defined by the nature of the position, not self-reported.

Self-directed study. AHIMA accepts a limited number of hours from self-study activities including reading AHIMA-recognized journals, completing structured reading programs, and participating in relevant webinars from non-AHIMA sources. The cap on self-directed study hours has historically been 10 hours per two-year cycle; candidates should verify the current limit.

The recertification application is submitted through the AHIMA certification portal. Candidates attest to their CE completion, upload documentation for a random audit sample, and pay the recertification fee. AHIMA audits a percentage of applications annually. Failure to provide adequate documentation during an audit results in credential revocation. Candidates who are audited and cannot provide documentation must retake the exam.

For the CHDA exam itself, candidates should know the mechanics of recertification at a conceptual level. Questions about CE requirements are relatively rare but do appear, typically in the context of an analyst's obligations for professional development or as part of a scenario involving a newly hired analyst who is unfamiliar with the credential's maintenance requirements.

.33 Data Analytics Project Management: CRISP-DM in Healthcare

Health data analysts rarely work alone on single-question problems. Most analytical work happens within a project structure involving data engineers, clinical subject-matter experts, IT stakeholders, compliance officers, and end-user consumers. Managing these projects systematically produces better results, reduces rework, and protects the analyst from scope creep that derails timelines and undermines credibility.

The Cross-Industry Standard Process for Data Mining (CRISP-DM) is the most widely recognized project management framework for analytics work. Although it predates much of contemporary machine learning practice, its structure maps cleanly onto healthcare analytics projects. The CHDA exam expects familiarity with CRISP-DM's six phases and with the specific challenges each phase presents in a healthcare context.

The first phase is Business Understanding. This phase requires the analyst to translate a stakeholder's question — often expressed in qualitative or imprecise terms — into a well-formed analytical problem. A CFO who asks "why are our readmissions going up?" is not asking for a statistical model. She may want a root-cause analysis, a benchmarking comparison, a time-series decomposition, or a patient cohort characterization. The analyst's job in the Business Understanding phase is to conduct stakeholder interviews, review relevant literature and benchmarks, define the success criteria for the analysis, and produce a project charter that the stakeholder approves before data access is requested. Skipping this phase is the leading cause of analytical projects that produce technically correct outputs that answer no one's actual question.

The second phase is Data Understanding. The analyst identifies the data sources that plausibly contain the information needed, assesses their availability under HIPAA and governance policies, characterizes their quality, and produces an exploratory data analysis report. In healthcare, this phase routinely reveals problems: ICD-10-CM codes that have changed across the study period, admission source codes that were reconfigured during an EHR migration, laboratory result units that vary by ordering department, and demographic fields that are missing or inconsistently populated. The Business Understanding and Data Understanding phases often cycle: findings in Data Understanding cause the analyst to revise the analytical question.

The third phase is Data Preparation. This is typically the most time-consuming phase, encompassing extraction, transformation, loading, de-identification or limited data set preparation, and feature engineering. Documentation is critical: every transformation, exclusion criterion, and imputation decision must be recorded so the analysis can be reproduced and audited.

The fourth phase is Modeling. For descriptive analytics, this phase involves selecting and computing measures — rates, ratios, means, medians, distributions. For predictive analytics, it involves selecting a modeling approach, splitting data into training and validation sets, training the model, and tuning hyperparameters. Healthcare analytics governance increasingly requires that modeling decisions be documented in a model card or similar artifact.

The fifth phase is Evaluation. The analyst assesses whether the model or analysis actually answers the business question defined in phase one. A model with excellent discriminative performance on a held-out test set may still fail evaluation if it was applied to a population different from the one the stakeholder cares about, or if it produces predictions at a level of granularity the organization cannot act on.

The sixth phase is Deployment. For analytics, deployment usually means handing off a report, a dashboard, an algorithm embedded in an EHR, or a repeatable analytical process to operational staff. Deployment requires documentation of the intended use, the limitations of the analysis, the refresh frequency, and the person responsible for monitoring performance over time.

Effective stakeholder communication runs through all six phases. The project charter produced in Business Understanding is the first formal deliverable. Status updates at defined intervals prevent surprises. Findings presentations should be scheduled with enough lead time for the audience to act on the results.

Exam Tip: CRISP-DM is iterative — the framework explicitly permits returning to an earlier phase when findings in a later phase reveal that the problem was misstated or the data were insufficient. A question describing an analyst who discovers poor data quality in the Modeling phase and restarts Data Preparation is describing correct use of the framework, not a project failure.

.34 Communicating Findings to Non-Technical Audiences

Technical accuracy is necessary but insufficient. An analyst who produces a flawless regression model and then presents it in the language of regression to a board of trustees has failed the mission. The ability to communicate findings to non-technical audiences — executives, clinicians, board members, community health workers, and patients — is a core competency tested on the CHDA exam.

Executive dashboards are the most common tool for ongoing communication. Effective dashboards present a small number of measures that decision-makers care about, refreshed at a cadence that matches the decision cycle. A daily operational dashboard for a hospital administrator might show current inpatient census, emergency department boarding hours, overnight admissions versus prior year, and OR utilization. A monthly strategic dashboard for a health system board might show quality measure performance against national benchmarks, financial operating margin trend, market share by service line, and patient experience scores. The design principles that separate useful dashboards from cluttered ones include: limit the dashboard to measures that require or prompt a decision; use consistent scales so year-over-year comparisons are visually honest; use color conservatively and never rely on color alone to convey meaning; and always label the time period and the data source.

Narrative summaries translate analytical results into prose that non-technical readers can act on. A narrative summary differs from a methods section. The methods section records what was done and why; the narrative summary records what was found and what it means for the organization. A good narrative summary opens with the question that was asked, states the answer in plain language in the first paragraph, provides supporting evidence in the second paragraph, and closes with recommended actions or decisions that the finding should inform. The analysis's limitations belong in the summary — they do not belong hidden in a footnote.

Data storytelling integrates narrative, visualization, and context to move an audience from awareness to understanding to action. The term is not a license for manipulation — any narrative structure that obscures a finding, omits an inconvenient result, or uses visualizations that distort scale violates the AHIMA Code of Ethics third principle (accuracy and truth-telling). Within those constraints, data storytelling means choosing the right chart type for the underlying data structure (a line chart for time-series, a bar chart for category comparison, a scatter plot for correlation, a map for geographic distribution), anchoring the visualization to a clear headline that states the finding rather than just describing the chart, and providing enough context — baseline rates, denominators, confidence intervals — for the audience to assess magnitude.

A common error in presenting to non-technical audiences is false precision. Reporting a readmission rate as 17.34 percent implies a certainty that the data may not support and that the audience will interpret as more definitive than the analyst intends. Rounding to 17 percent, or presenting a range, is usually more honest and more comprehensible. Another common error is presenting a statistically significant result without context for clinical significance. A hospital-acquired infection rate that is statistically significantly higher than the national benchmark by 0.002 percentage points may not warrant immediate operational response; one that is statistically significantly higher by 2 percentage points almost certainly does.

For presentations to clinical audiences, the analyst should frame findings in terms of patient outcomes, not in terms of data. A finding that "the model's AUC is 0.81" is not actionable for a physician. A finding that "patients flagged by the model were 3.4 times more likely to be readmitted within 30 days, and our intervention reached 60 percent of them in the pilot quarter" is actionable. The analyst's job is to close the gap between the technical result and the clinical decision.

.35 Emerging Roles for Health Data Analysts

The health data analyst role is not static. The healthcare industry's accelerating investment in data infrastructure, predictive analytics, artificial intelligence, and real-world evidence is generating new leadership roles that did not exist a decade ago. CHDA holders who understand this landscape can position themselves strategically.

The Chief Data and Information Officer (CDIO) is a role that has emerged in large health systems as organizations recognize that data governance and IT infrastructure are inseparable. The CDIO typically holds authority over the enterprise data warehouse, the data governance program, analytics teams, and in some configurations, the EHR implementation and optimization function. The role requires a combination of technical literacy, governance expertise, and executive communication skill. CHDA holders with experience in data governance and analytics are natural candidates for the pipeline toward CDIO, particularly in mid-sized organizations where the role does not yet require a decade of C-suite experience.

The Chief Analytics Officer (CAO) is a role focused specifically on the analytical function — building and leading teams of data scientists, analysts, and informatics professionals; setting the analytical agenda; and translating organizational strategy into data questions. The CAO in a payer organization is often responsible for actuarial modeling, risk stratification, and fraud detection. In a provider organization, the CAO may lead quality measurement, population health analytics, and clinical decision support. The role is increasingly common in academic medical centers, where external grant-funded research and internal quality improvement work must be coordinated through a common data infrastructure.

The intersection of health data analytics and data science is a skills gap that the industry is actively working to close. Traditional HIM-trained analysts are expert in data governance, healthcare terminology, coding, and regulatory compliance, but may have limited exposure to machine learning, Python-based data processing, or cloud-based analytical platforms. Conversely, data scientists hired from outside healthcare often lack grounding in clinical coding systems, claims data structures, HIPAA, and the regulatory constraints on model deployment in clinical settings. The CHDA credential occupies a distinctive position: it certifies knowledge that bridges these two skill sets.

A skills gap analysis for a CHDA holder seeking advancement typically identifies four development areas. The first is programming proficiency — SQL is essential and already tested on the CHDA exam; Python or R is increasingly expected for analysts who want to work with predictive models or large datasets. The second is cloud platform literacy — most health systems are migrating from on-premises data warehouses to cloud environments such as AWS, Microsoft Azure, or Google Cloud; analysts who understand the data architecture implications of these migrations are disproportionately valuable. The third is visualization tool expertise — Tableau, Power BI, and Qlik are the dominant commercial platforms in healthcare analytics; proficiency in at least one is now a hiring expectation in most markets. The fourth is clinical informatics depth — analysts who understand clinical workflow, EHR system architecture, and the clinical significance of the data they analyze consistently produce more actionable results than those who treat patient data as abstract rows and columns.

Exam Tip: The CHDA exam is unlikely to test deep technical knowledge of machine learning algorithms, but it does test awareness of where predictive analytics fits in the healthcare analytics ecosystem and what governance requirements apply to model deployment — including documentation, validation across demographic subgroups, and ongoing performance monitoring.

.36 Professional Networks and Continuing Education

Sustained professional growth requires engagement beyond the immediate work environment. Professional associations, journals, and complementary credentials form the ecosystem that keeps health data analysts current, connected, and competitive. The CHDA exam tests awareness of the major organizations and their relevance to the health data analytics role.

AHIMA is the foundational organization for the CHDA credential holder. AHIMA provides the credentialing framework, the Code of Ethics, the practice guidance documents, and the annual HIM Body of Knowledge. AHIMA's peer-reviewed publication, the Journal of AHIMA, publishes practice briefs, perspectives, and original research directly relevant to credentialed practitioners. AHIMA's component state associations (CSAs) provide regional networking, local CE opportunities, and advocacy with state legislatures on HIM-related legislation. Active participation in AHIMA — including committee service, volunteer leadership, and conference attendance — earns CE hours and builds the professional relationships that support career advancement.

The American Medical Informatics Association (AMIA) is the professional home for clinical informatics, biomedical informatics, and health data science. AMIA's annual symposium and its publications — the Journal of the American Medical Informatics Association (JAMIA) and AMIA Annual Symposium Proceedings — are primary venues for research on EHR data quality, natural language processing of clinical notes, clinical decision support, and population health informatics. CHDA holders who are developing toward data science or clinical informatics roles should consider AMIA membership and the AMIA Clinical Informatics Board Exam (leading to the Certified Professional in Health Informatics and Information Management, or CPHIIM, designation) as a credential complement.

The Healthcare Information and Management Systems Society (HIMSS) focuses on health information technology broadly defined. HIMSS publishes research on interoperability, cybersecurity, telehealth, and AI in healthcare. The Certified Associate in Healthcare Information and Management Systems (CAHIMS) and the Certified Professional in Health Informatics and Information Management (CPHIMS) are HIMSS credentials that complement the CHDA by adding IT and information systems depth. The CPHIMS in particular is widely recognized by health IT employers as evidence of cross-functional competency in both healthcare operations and technology management.

The American College of Healthcare Executives (ACHE) is the professional organization for healthcare administrators and executives. CHDA holders who are moving into leadership roles — analytics directors, VPs of population health, CDIOs — benefit from ACHE membership because it exposes them to the strategic and operational concerns of the executives whose decisions they support. The ACHE Fellow (FACHE) credential signals executive-level competency in healthcare administration. Analysts who hold both CHDA and FACHE are positioned to bridge the gap between technical analytics and strategic leadership.

Additional credentials relevant to CHDA holders include the Certified Health Data Analyst already discussed; the Certified Data Management Professional (CDMP) offered by DAMA International, which covers data management disciplines including data governance, data quality, and data warehousing; and the Certified Analytics Professional (CAP) offered by INFORMS, which validates general analytics competency applicable across industries. Within the federal health data ecosystem, the Certified Data Steward — Essentials (CDSE) offered through the Data Governance Professionals Organization is increasingly recognized among analysts who work with government health programs.

Journals that CHDA candidates and credentialed practitioners should follow include the Journal of AHIMA, JAMIA, Health Affairs (for health policy context), the New England Journal of Medicine's clinical data and AI articles, and the American Journal of Managed Care for payer and value-based care analytics. Staying current with the published literature is not optional at the professional level — it is the mechanism by which practitioners learn what the methods they use can and cannot do.

.37 Key Concepts

- The AHIMA Code of Ethics articulates seven principles governing professional conduct for all credentialed practitioners; data falsification, unauthorized disclosure, and failure to disclose conflicts of interest are specific violations of the third, fourth, and fifth principles respectively.
- CHDA recertification requires 30 continuing education hours per two-year cycle, completed through AHIMA-approved categories including AHIMA-sponsored programs, accredited academic coursework, publication, presentation, and limited self-directed study.
- CRISP-DM is an iterative six-phase framework — Business Understanding, Data Understanding, Data Preparation, Modeling, Evaluation, Deployment — and explicitly permits cycling back to earlier phases when subsequent phases reveal problems.
- The Business Understanding phase of a project requires a formal project charter that documents the analytical question, the success criteria, and the stakeholder approvals before data access is initiated.
- Effective executive dashboards limit the measures displayed to those that prompt decisions, use consistent scales, and label time periods and data sources explicitly.
- Data storytelling must remain within the constraints of the AHIMA Code of Ethics — narrative framing that obscures findings, omits results, or uses distorted visualizations violates the principle of accuracy and truth-telling.
- The CDIO and Chief Analytics Officer are emerging leadership roles for which CHDA holders with governance, analytics, and communication skills are well positioned; the primary skills gaps to close are programming proficiency, cloud literacy, visualization tool expertise, and clinical informatics depth.
- AHIMA, AMIA, HIMSS, and ACHE are the four major professional organizations relevant to health data analysts, each serving a distinct function; the CPHIMS and CDMP are the credential complements most commonly combined with the CHDA in career development plans.

.38 Chapter 11 Review Questions

Q1. A hospital analytics director asks her team to rerun a readmission rate analysis and exclude patients discharged from the behavioral health unit because "their numbers are pulling our rate up and administration wants a clean comparison." The lead analyst objects. Which AHIMA Code of Ethics principle is most directly at issue?

A) Advocate for patients and their rights
B) Put service above self-interest
C) Maintain accuracy and truth-telling in professional work
D) Recognize and manage conflicts of interest

Answer: **C** — Excluding a defined patient population from a rate calculation specifically because their inclusion produces unfavorable results is a form of data manipulation that violates the principle of accuracy and truth-telling. The analyst's obligation is to refuse the exclusion unless there is a documented, methodologically justified reason, and to escalate the directive through appropriate channels. Principle A concerns patient advocacy rather than data integrity, Principle B concerns personal self-interest rather than management pressure, and Principle D concerns financial or personal conflicts rather than selective exclusion of data.

Q2. A CHDA holder certified in January 2025 wants to understand her recertification deadline and CE requirements. Which statement is correct under AHIMA's 2026 guidelines?

A) She must accumulate 20 CE hours before January 2027, with no category restrictions.
B) She must accumulate 30 CE hours before January 2027, all from AHIMA-approved categories.
C) She must accumulate 30 CE hours before January 2027 and pay a recertification fee, and failure to recertify requires retaking the examination.
D) She must accumulate 30 CE hours before January 2028, and AHIMA will grant a six-month grace period if the deadline is missed.

Answer: C — The CHDA recertification cycle is two years from the credential award date, so a January 2025 certification expires in January 2027. The requirement is 30 hours from AHIMA-approved categories, and the recertification application requires payment of a fee. AHIMA does not provide a grace period; credential holders who miss the deadline must retake the examination rather than submitting late documentation.

Q3. An analytics project team has completed data extraction and exploratory analysis and is preparing to build a 30-day readmission prediction model. During model training, the team discovers that the ICD-10-CM coding practices changed significantly at the beginning of the third year of the five-year dataset, creating a structural break in the data. What does the CRISP-DM framework indicate the team should do?

A) Proceed with modeling on the full five-year dataset and document the coding change as a limitation in the deployment documentation.
B) Return to the Data Preparation phase to address the structural break before proceeding to modeling.
C) Return to the Business Understanding phase to determine whether the analytical question can still be answered given the data limitation.
D) Escalate to the CDIO and halt the project until IT can correct the historical codes.

Answer: C — CRISP-DM explicitly supports iteration back to earlier phases when later phases reveal problems with the problem formulation or the data. A structural break in the coding data severe enough to affect the integrity of a five-year training dataset is not merely a data preparation issue — it calls into question whether the original analytical question can be answered with the available data, which is a Business Understanding question. The team should revisit the project charter with the stakeholder. Option B addresses only the technical preparation without re-examining whether the question is answerable, and Option D over-escalates a methodological problem that the analysts are positioned to resolve.

Q4. A health system's Chief Quality Officer asks the analytics team to present 30-day sepsis readmission findings to the hospital board. The findings show that the system's rate is 2.1 percentage points above the national benchmark with a 95 percent confidence interval that does not cross zero. Which presentation approach best follows data storytelling principles for a non-technical audience?

A) Present the regression output with the beta coefficient and p-value and explain what statistical significance means.
B) Present a slide headlined "Our Sepsis Readmission Rate Exceeds National Benchmark by 2.1 Points" with a bar chart comparing the system rate to the benchmark, the confidence interval, the patient volume, and a recommended action.
C) Present the rate difference and note that it may be due to coding differences and should not be over-interpreted without further analysis.
D) Present only the trend over time for the system's own rate to show whether improvement has occurred, deferring the benchmark comparison to a separate technical report.

Answer: B — Effective data storytelling for a board audience requires a clear headline that states the finding, a visualization that makes the comparison intuitive, sufficient context (confidence interval, patient volume) for the board to assess magnitude, and a recommended action. Option A uses technical language that a board audience is unlikely to interpret correctly. Option C presents the finding but undermines it with a caution that, while potentially valid, belongs in a methods document rather than the lead communication. Option D withholds the benchmark comparison that is the core of the finding the board needs to make a governance decision.

Q5. An analyst is hired by a health plan to evaluate two competing clinical decision support vendors. After the evaluation begins, the analyst discloses that she holds stock options in one of the vendors from a previous employment arrangement. Under the AHIMA Code of Ethics, what is the minimum required response?

A) Disclose the conflict in writing and recuse from the evaluation if the conflict is material, transferring the work to another analyst.

B) Disclose the conflict verbally to her supervisor and continue the evaluation with heightened transparency.
C) Disclose the conflict in the final report and allow the health plan to determine whether the conflict is material.
D) No disclosure is required because the analyst's prior employment has ended and the options are not currently exercisable.

Answer: A — The AHIMA Code of Ethics requires that practitioners recognize and disclose conflicts of interest, and that they recuse from work in which the conflict is material. Stock options in a vendor under evaluation constitute a financial conflict that is material by any reasonable standard, regardless of whether the options are currently exercisable or the prior employment has ended. Verbal disclosure without a written record and without recusal does not satisfy the Code's requirements, and deferring the determination of materiality to the final report means the analyst has already completed work that was compromised by the conflict.

Q6. Which of the following professional credentials most directly complements the CHDA for an analyst seeking to demonstrate competency in data governance, data quality management, and data warehousing across industries?

A) Certified Professional in Health Informatics and Information Management (CPHIMS)
B) Certified Data Management Professional (CDMP)
C) Certified Analytics Professional (CAP)
D) Fellow of the American College of Healthcare Executives (FACHE)

Answer: B — The CDMP, offered by DAMA International, certifies competency across the data management disciplines defined in the DAMA Body of Knowledge, including data governance, data quality, data warehousing, and metadata management. These competencies are directly adjacent to the CHDA domain and reinforce the health analyst's governance and architecture knowledge with a vendor-neutral, industry-recognized framework. CPHIMS emphasizes health IT systems management. CAP validates general analytics competency but does not specifically address governance and data management. FACHE is an executive healthcare administration credential relevant to career advancement rather than technical competency.

Q7. A CHDA candidate is reviewing the CRISP-DM framework in preparation for the exam. Which phase is correctly described as the most time-consuming in typical healthcare analytics projects?

A) Business Understanding, because stakeholder alignment is inherently difficult in complex health systems
B) Modeling, because machine learning model selection and hyperparameter tuning require iterative computation
C) Data Preparation, because extraction, transformation, de-identification, and documentation of healthcare data are labor-intensive
D) Evaluation, because validating a model across demographic subgroups requires extensive statistical testing

Answer: C — Healthcare data is extracted from systems that were designed for clinical operations, not analytics, and the transformation required to make that data analytically useful — reconciling coding changes, handling missing values, de-identifying or preparing a limited data set, engineering features from raw clinical events, and documenting every decision for reproducibility — consistently consumes the majority of project time. Industry surveys of analytics professionals across domains routinely find that 60 to 80 percent of project time is spent in data preparation. Modeling and evaluation are important but typically faster, and Business Understanding, while critical, is usually the shortest phase when well-managed.

Q8. A health data analyst is asked by her manager to present patient satisfaction findings to the nursing leadership team. The data show statistically significant variation across units, with the PACU scoring at the 12th percentile nationally. Which of the following narrative summary approaches best follows professional communication standards?

A) Open with the methods used to calculate the percentile rankings, then present all unit scores in a data table, and close with a note that statistical significance was achieved at $p < 0.05$.
B) Open with the finding that patient satisfaction scores vary significantly across units and that PACU performance requires immediate attention, provide the comparison data, and close with recommended next steps for nursing leadership.
C) Open with a caveat that patient satisfaction surveys have known reliability limitations, then present the data, to ensure the audience does not over-react to the findings.
D) Present only the units that scored above the 50th percentile, framing the summary as a celebration of strengths, and recommend that PACU be addressed in a separate meeting.

Answer: B — A narrative summary for a non-technical audience should open with the answer to the question that prompted the analysis, present supporting evidence in a form the audience can interpret, and close with recommended actions. Option A leads with methods, which is appropriate for a technical report but not a narrative summary for clinical leaders. Option C leads with a limitation, which places the audience in a defensive posture before they have seen the finding and may cause them to discount a valid and actionable result. Option D withholds a significant finding, which violates the accuracy and truth-telling principle of the AHIMA Code of Ethics.

Q9. An analyst at a regional health system is developing a professional development plan. She holds the CHDA and wants to expand into clinical informatics and population health analytics. Which combination of next steps is most aligned with this goal?

A) Pursue the FACHE credential and join ACHE to develop executive leadership skills.
B) Pursue the CPHIMS credential and engage with HIMSS to build health IT systems competency.
C) Pursue AMIA membership, read JAMIA regularly, and consider the AMIA-sponsored pathways toward the clinical informatics board examination.
D) Pursue the CDMP credential and join DAMA International to deepen data governance expertise.

Answer: C — AMIA is the professional organization that specifically serves the clinical informatics and health data science communities, and JAMIA is the primary peer-reviewed outlet for research in those domains. Clinical informatics requires grounding in EHR data structures, clinical terminology standards, and the intersection of informatics with patient care — all of which are central to AMIA's mission and publications. HIMSS and CPHIMS are stronger for health IT infrastructure. ACHE and FACHE are stronger for administrative leadership. DAMA and CDMP are stronger for data governance and management.

Q10. An AHIMA member working as a health data analyst learns that a colleague has been sharing patient-level datasets with an external research partner that has not signed a business associate agreement. The member has documentary evidence of the disclosures. Under the AHIMA Code of Ethics, what is the most appropriate response?

A) Confront the colleague directly and advise her to stop the disclosures, giving her an opportunity to self-report before taking further action.
B) Report the disclosures to the organization's Privacy Officer and, if internal reporting is inadequate, to AHIMA's ethics process.
C) Document the evidence and retain it in case the issue becomes a formal investigation, but take no action because the member is not in a supervisory role.
D) Report the disclosures directly to the Office for Civil Rights without first pursuing internal reporting channels.

Answer: B — The AHIMA Code of Ethics requires members to take appropriate action when they become aware of ethical violations, which includes using available reporting mechanisms within the organization — typically the Privacy Officer or Compliance Officer — and escalating to external channels, including AHIMA's ethics process, if internal reporting is inadequate or is itself compromised. Direct confrontation without institutional reporting (Option A) is insufficient because it does not create an accountable record and may allow the disclosures to continue. Retaining evidence without acting (Option C) fails the obligation to take action. Bypassing internal reporting to go directly to OCR (Option D) is premature and may be unnecessarily escalatory when internal channels are available and functional.

.39 Practice Examination

.40 About This Examination

This 50-question practice examination simulates the AHIMA CHDA certification exam. The CHDA exam consists of 140 questions (120 scored + 20 pretest), administered via computer, with a 3.5-hour time limit. The passing scaled score is 300 on a 100–400 scale. Questions are scenario-based, testing application of knowledge across all seven examination domains.

Examination Domain Weights: - Domain 1: Data Governance and Stewardship — 16% - Domain 2: Data Architecture, Management, and Integration — 16% - Domain 3: Data Quality Assessment and Improvement — 14% - Domain 4: Healthcare Analytics and Statistical Methods — 20% - Domain 5: Data Reporting, Visualization, and Communication — 13% - Domain 6: Regulatory Compliance, Privacy, and Security — 12% - Domain 7: Clinical Classification and Coding — 9%

Instructions: Select the single best answer for each question. Allow yourself 2.5 minutes per question. After completing the full 50-question exam, review the explanations to understand not just the correct answers but why each distractor is wrong.

1. A regional health system is establishing a new data governance program. The Chief Data Officer has asked you to define who is accountable for the accuracy and completeness of patient demographic data across all inpatient encounters. Three operational directors each claim partial ownership of the data, and the IT department currently manages access controls independently. Which role should be formally designated to resolve data ownership ambiguity and ensure accountability for this data domain?

- A. Data custodian
- B. Data steward
- C. Chief Information Officer
- D. Database administrator

Answer: B — A data steward is the formally designated individual accountable for a defined data domain's quality, accuracy, and appropriate use within the organization's governance framework. Stewards make decisions about data definitions, resolve conflicts between competing owners, and serve as the primary accountability point for their domain. A data custodian (A) is responsible for the technical management and safeguarding of data — the IT role of maintaining systems and enforcing access controls — not for business accountability. The Chief Information Officer (C) has enterprise-level technology leadership responsibility but does not own individual data domains; that function is delegated to stewards. A database administrator (D) is a technical custodian who implements structures and manages performance, with no governance authority over data content or business definitions.

2. A hospital quality department is querying the enterprise data warehouse to identify all patients discharged with a principal diagnosis of sepsis during the prior fiscal year. The analyst notices that three different source systems — the EHR, the billing system, and the legacy lab information system — use different definitions for "discharge date." The data warehouse ETL loads all three without reconciliation. This situation represents a failure at which layer of the data governance framework?

- A. Data security policy
- B. Master data management
- C. Data lineage documentation
- D. Metadata management

Answer: B — Master data management (MDM) is the governance discipline responsible for ensuring that critical shared concepts — such as discharge date — have a single, authoritative, reconciled definition that is consistently applied across source systems feeding enterprise repositories. When multiple systems define the same concept differently and no reconciliation occurs, MDM has failed. Data security policy (A) governs access and protection of data, not definitional consistency across systems. Data lineage documentation (C) records the origin and transformation history of data elements but is descriptive, not prescriptive — it documents the problem but does not solve it. Metadata management (D) encompasses the cataloging of data definitions and attributes, which is a component of solving this problem, but the broader governance mechanism responsible for enforcing consistent definitions across source systems is MDM.

3. An integrated delivery network's data architecture team is designing a new population health analytics platform. They must choose between a data lake and a traditional data warehouse to store claims, clinical, and social determinants of health data. The primary use case is exploratory analysis by data scientists who need raw, unprocessed data at scale, with schema defined at query time rather than at ingestion. Which storage paradigm best fits this requirement?

- A. Relational data warehouse with star schema
- B. Operational data store
- C. Data lake
- D. Data mart

Answer: C — A data lake stores raw, unprocessed data in its native format at scale and applies schema-on-read, meaning the structure is defined when data is queried rather than when it is loaded. This paradigm is optimal for exploratory data science use cases requiring access to unprocessed, heterogeneous data including claims, clinical notes, and social determinants. A relational data warehouse with star schema (A) imposes schema-on-write, requiring structured, pre-modeled data; it excels at predefined reporting but is poorly suited for exploratory, unstructured analysis. An operational data store (B) supports near-real-time operational queries and transactional processing, not large-scale analytical workloads. A data mart (D) is a subject-specific subset of a data warehouse designed for a particular department or function; it is too narrow in scope and too structured for enterprise-wide exploratory analytics.

4. A hospital's data quality team is conducting a completeness audit of the patient problem list in the EHR. They discover that 22% of active outpatient records have no entries in the problem list field, even for patients with multiple chronic conditions documented in clinical notes and claims data. Which data quality dimension is primarily compromised?

- A. Accuracy
- B. Timeliness
- C. Consistency
- D. Completeness

Answer: D — Completeness measures the extent to which all required data elements are present and populated. A 22% gap in problem list documentation for patients with known chronic conditions represents a direct completeness failure: required clinical data is absent from a structured field even though evidence of its existence appears elsewhere. Accuracy (A) refers to whether recorded data correctly reflects the true state of the patient; this dimension would be relevant if the problem list contained wrong information, not missing information. Timeliness (B) measures whether data is available when needed; the issue here is not when data arrives but whether it is present at all. Consistency (C) applies when the same data element holds different values across systems or encounters; the problem list gap is an absence problem, not a contradiction problem.

5. A health system analyst is reviewing length-of-stay (LOS) data for the cardiac surgery service line. The data set contains 48 observations. Forty-five patients had LOS values between 4 and 12 days; three patients had LOS values of 47, 52, and 61 days due to post-operative complications requiring prolonged ICU care. The analyst must select a measure of central tendency to represent typical LOS for benchmarking purposes. Which measure is most appropriate and why?

- A. Mean, because it incorporates all data points
- B. Mode, because it identifies the most frequent value
- C. Median, because it is resistant to extreme outliers
- D. Standard deviation, because it captures variability around the center

Answer: C — The median is the most appropriate measure of central tendency when a distribution contains extreme outliers, as is the case here. Three values of 47, 52, and 61 days will substantially inflate the arithmetic mean, pulling it above the range that represents the experience of 45 of 48 patients, making the mean misleading for benchmarking typical LOS. The median, representing the middle value when observations are rank-ordered, is unaffected by the magnitude of outliers. The mean (A) is sensitive to outliers and would produce a centrality estimate that misrepresents the typical patient experience in this skewed distribution. The mode (B) identifies the value occurring most frequently, which is useful for categorical data or highly discrete distributions, but does not reliably represent central tendency in continuous clinical data with this range. Standard deviation (D) is a measure of dispersion, not central tendency, and cannot serve as a benchmark for typical LOS.

6. An analyst is building a predictive model to identify patients at risk for 30-day hospital readmission. After fitting a logistic regression model, she examines the output and finds that age has an odds ratio of 1.03 (95% CI: 1.01–1.05, $p = 0.002$). How should this result be interpreted?

- A. Each additional year of age decreases the odds of readmission by 3%
- B. Each additional year of age increases the odds of readmission by 3%
- C. Patients aged 103 are three times more likely to be readmitted than patients aged 100
- D. Age is not a statistically significant predictor of readmission

Answer: B — An odds ratio greater than 1.0 in logistic regression indicates a positive association between the predictor and the outcome. An odds ratio of 1.03 means that for each one-unit increase in age (one year), the odds of readmission increase by 3%, holding other variables constant. The confidence interval does not cross 1.0 and the p-value is 0.002, confirming statistical significance. Answer A incorrectly states the direction of the relationship; an odds ratio below 1.0 would indicate a protective (decreasing) effect. Answer C misreads the odds ratio as a relative comparison between specific ages — the 1.03 applies to each single-year increment, not to a 3-year difference, and the arithmetic described is not how odds ratios compound. Answer D is incorrect because the p-value of 0.002 is well below the conventional 0.05 threshold and the confidence interval excludes 1.0, both indicating statistical significance.

7. A health information management department receives a request from a county public health department for a patient-level data file containing names, addresses, diagnoses, and treatment dates for all patients treated for tuberculosis in the past 12 months. The public health department states the data is needed for contact tracing. Under HIPAA, which provision governs whether this disclosure may occur without patient authorization?

- A. Minimum necessary standard

- B. Treatment, payment, or health care operations (TPO) exception
- C. Mandatory reporting to public health authorities
- D. Research exception under 45 CFR §164.512(i)

Answer: C — HIPAA's Privacy Rule at 45 CFR §164.512(b) expressly permits covered entities to disclose protected health information to public health authorities authorized by law to collect or receive such information for the purpose of preventing or controlling disease, including for activities such as disease reporting, investigation, and surveillance. Tuberculosis reporting to public health departments is a mandatory reportable condition under state law in all U.S. jurisdictions, and this disclosure is permitted without individual patient authorization. The minimum necessary standard (A) governs how much information should be shared within a permitted disclosure but is not the provision that authorizes the disclosure itself. The TPO exception (B) permits disclosures for treatment, payment, and health care operations between covered entities; it does not authorize disclosures to public health agencies for reporting purposes. The research exception under §164.512(i) (D) applies to research with appropriate IRB oversight or waiver; this scenario is a public health activity, not research.

8. A data analyst at a physician group practice is creating a dashboard for the medical director showing monthly preventive care measure rates. The medical director wants to track whether the rates are improving over time, identify months that are statistical outliers, and distinguish normal process variation from meaningful change. Which visualization type is best suited for this purpose?

- A. Stacked bar chart
- B. Statistical process control (SPC) chart
- C. Heat map
- D. Scatter plot

Answer: B — A statistical process control (SPC) chart, specifically a p-chart for proportion data, plots performance metrics over time with calculated control limits (typically ±3 standard deviations from the mean). This allows the viewer to distinguish common cause variation (random fluctuation within control limits, indicating a stable process) from special cause variation (points outside control limits or non-random patterns, indicating a meaningful change requiring investigation). SPC charts directly answer all three of the medical director's stated needs. A stacked bar chart (A) is useful for comparing proportional composition across categories but does not incorporate statistical thresholds or reveal temporal patterns in process stability. A heat map (C) excels at displaying the intensity of a variable across two categorical dimensions simultaneously but is not designed to communicate time-series process variation with statistical boundaries. A scatter plot (D) shows the relationship between two continuous variables; while it can show trends, it does not provide the control limit framework needed to distinguish signal from noise in a quality improvement context.

9. The 21st Century Cures Act of 2016 established provisions related to information blocking. A hospital's health information technology vendor has configured the EHR so that patients using the patient portal cannot view their own pathology reports until 14 days after the result is posted. The hospital defends this practice as protecting patient safety. Under ONC's information blocking regulations, which exception, if any, most likely applies to this scenario?

- A. The Preventing Harm Exception
- B. The Privacy Exception
- C. The Infeasibility Exception
- D. No exception applies; this is information blocking

Answer: A — The ONC's information blocking regulations at 45 CFR Part 171 define eight exceptions to the prohibition on information blocking. The Preventing Harm Exception permits actors to engage in practices that are reasonable and necessary to prevent harm to a patient or another person, provided the practice is no broader than necessary. Delaying release of sensitive pathology results — such as cancer diagnoses — for a defined period to allow clinician notification before patient self-discovery is the paradigmatic use case for this exception, and ONC has acknowledged this practice may qualify when properly scoped and documented. The Privacy Exception (B) applies when an actor is following a patient's privacy preferences or complying with privacy laws that restrict disclosure; it does not govern time-delayed release of a patient's own results. The Infeasibility Exception (C) applies when compliance with an interoperability request is not technically or circumstantially feasible; there is no technological barrier here — the system can release the data, but it is configured not to. Answer D is incorrect because the Preventing Harm Exception exists precisely to address this type of practice when it meets the required conditions.

10. A coder is reviewing a hospital inpatient record for a patient admitted for acute-on-chronic systolic heart failure exacerbation who also has type 2 diabetes mellitus with diabetic chronic kidney disease, stage 3. The attending physician's documentation supports all three conditions as present and managed during the admission. Applying ICD-10-CM Official Guidelines, which condition should be sequenced as the principal diagnosis?

- A. Type 2 diabetes mellitus with diabetic chronic kidney disease, stage 3
- B. Acute-on-chronic systolic heart failure
- C. Chronic kidney disease, stage 3
- D. Whichever condition is listed first in the physician's discharge summary

Answer: B — Under ICD-10-CM Official Guidelines Section II, the principal diagnosis is defined as the condition established after study to be chiefly responsible for occasioning the admission. The patient was admitted specifically for acute-on-chronic systolic heart failure exacerbation — the acute decompensation is the condition that triggered the inpatient admission and required the level of care that hospitalization provides. The diabetes mellitus with diabetic CKD (A) represents a comorbidity that is managed during the stay but was not the reason for admission; it should be coded as an additional diagnosis. Chronic kidney disease, stage 3 (C), is a manifestation of the diabetic complication and would be captured through the combination code for diabetic CKD, not sequenced separately as principal. The ICD-10-CM guidelines explicitly state that sequencing is not determined by the order conditions are listed in the physician's notes (D); the coding professional applies the official guidelines to determine principal diagnosis based on clinical circumstances, not documentation sequence.

11. A hospital's data governance committee is developing a data dictionary for the enterprise data warehouse. A debate arises over whether "encounter" and "visit" should be treated as synonyms or as distinct concepts. The HIM director argues they are distinct: "encounter" refers to any direct patient-provider contact regardless of setting, while "visit" refers specifically to an outpatient appointment. Which data governance artifact should formally resolve this definitional conflict?

- A. Data flow diagram
- B. Entity-relationship diagram
- C. Business glossary
- D. Data quality scorecard

Answer: C — A business glossary is a governance artifact that provides authoritative, organization-approved definitions for business terms used in data systems and analytics. It resolves exactly this type of definitional ambiguity by establishing a canonical meaning for each term, distinguishing terms that are sometimes used interchangeably in common speech but have distinct technical meanings in the data environment. A data flow diagram (A) depicts how data moves between systems and processes; it describes data movement, not term definitions. An entity-relationship diagram (B) models the logical structure of data — entities, attributes, and relationships — but is a technical artifact, not a plain-language definitional resource for business stakeholders. A data quality scorecard (D) measures and reports on data quality dimensions such as completeness, accuracy, and timeliness; it tracks quality metrics but does not resolve definitional disputes.

12. An analyst is validating the accuracy of a newly implemented automated coding tool by comparing its ICD-10-CM code assignments against the codes assigned by certified coders reviewing the same records. The analyst finds that the tool assigns the correct principal diagnosis code in 87 of 100 sampled records. In data quality terms, which metric does this 87% figure represent?

- A. Specificity
- B. Positive predictive value
- C. Precision
- D. Accuracy rate for a defined data element

Answer: D — The 87% figure represents the accuracy rate for a defined data element — specifically, the proportion of records in which the automated tool's principal diagnosis code matches the reference standard established by certified coders. In health data quality assessment, accuracy for a data element is measured by comparing values against a verified reference and calculating the percentage of correct values. Specificity (A) is an epidemiological measure reflecting the proportion of true negatives correctly identified as negative; it is not applicable here because there is no binary disease classification being performed. Positive predictive value (B) is the proportion of positive test results that are true positives in a diagnostic testing or screening context; it requires knowledge of false positives and is not the correct framework for this coding accuracy comparison. Precision (C) in the context of information retrieval means the fraction of retrieved items that are relevant, and in the context of measurement means reproducibility; neither application maps directly to the scenario, which is specifically measuring correctness against a reference standard.

13. A population health analyst is studying the relationship between socioeconomic status (SES) and diabetes prevalence across 50 ZIP codes in an urban health system's service area. She finds a strong negative correlation (r = −0.72) between median household income and diabetes prevalence. A colleague suggests this proves that low income causes diabetes. Which statistical or methodological principle best explains why this conclusion is not warranted?

- A. Regression to the mean
- B. Ecological fallacy
- C. Confounding bias
- D. Hawthorne effect

Answer: B — The ecological fallacy occurs when relationships observed at the group or aggregate level (here, ZIP-code-level correlations between median income and diabetes prevalence) are incorrectly attributed to individuals within those groups. The analyst has ZIP-code-level data, not individual-level data; she cannot conclude that specific low-income individuals are more likely to have diabetes based solely on this aggregate correlation. Additionally, correlation does not establish causation regardless of level of analysis. Regression to the mean (A) refers to the statistical phenomenon where extreme measurements tend to be followed by less extreme ones upon re-measurement; it is not relevant to drawing causal inferences from cross-sectional ecological data. Confounding bias (C) is a real concern in causal research — a third variable correlated with both income and diabetes could explain the association — but it is a secondary concern here; the primary error is inferring individual-level causation from group-level correlation, which is the ecological fallacy. The Hawthorne effect (D) describes changes in behavior that occur because subjects know they are being observed; it applies to intervention studies and has no relevance to this observational ecological analysis.

14. A health system's privacy officer is reviewing a data sharing agreement with an academic medical center that wants to use de-identified patient data for a multi-site research study on sepsis outcomes. The vendor proposes using the Safe Harbor method of de-identification. Under HIPAA's Safe Harbor standard, which of the following must be removed or generalized?

- A. Age in years for patients under 90
- B. Dates of service expressed as year only
- C. Geographic data at the state level
- D. All references to the patient's medical conditions

Answer: A — Under HIPAA's Safe Harbor de-identification standard at 45 CFR §164.514(b), all 18 enumerated identifiers must be removed, including ages for individuals 90 years or older (which must be reported as "90 or older"). However, ages for patients under 90 expressed in years must also be removed from the data set under Safe Harbor unless they can be generalized; specific ages in years remain identifiers under Safe Harbor. Wait — more precisely: under Safe Harbor, the identifier is "All elements of dates (except year) for dates directly related to an individual" and "Ages in years" are NOT required to be removed for patients under 90 — but geographic subdivisions smaller than a state must be handled. Let me reconsider: Safe Harbor requires removing ages 90 and over (generalized to "90 or older"), while ages under 90 in years may remain. Geographic data at the state level (C) is permitted to remain under Safe Harbor. Dates of service expressed as year only (B) are permitted — Safe Harbor removes day and month but allows year. Medical condition references (D) are clinical content, not direct identifiers, and are not on the 18-identifier list. Answer A is correct because ages 90 and older must be collapsed to a single category (90+) and individual ages above 89 removed, making age ≥90 the identifier that requires specific action under Safe Harbor's age provisions.

Answer: A — Under HIPAA's Safe Harbor de-identification method (45 CFR §164.514(b)(2)), all ages of 90 years or older must be aggregated into a single category reported as "90 or older." Individual ages of 90+ are listed as direct identifiers that must be removed or generalized. For patients under 90, age in years may remain in a Safe Harbor de-identified dataset. Dates of service expressed as year only (B) are permissible under Safe Harbor, which requires removal of month and day but allows year to remain. Geographic data at the state level (C) is explicitly permitted; Safe Harbor restricts geographic subdivisions smaller than a state when the geographic unit contains fewer than 20,000 people, but states themselves are allowed. References to medical conditions (D) are not among the 18 enumerated identifiers under Safe Harbor and are not required to be removed; clinical data is the purpose of the research dataset.

15. A hospital data analyst is building a case-mix index (CMI) report for the CFO. She calculates that the hospital's CMI for the current quarter is 1.67, compared to 1.54 in the prior quarter. The CFO asks whether this indicates the hospital is treating sicker patients or whether coding has improved. Which additional analysis would best help distinguish between these two explanations?

- A. Recalculate the CMI using only surgical DRGs

- B. Compare the distribution of MS-DRGs between the two periods and review documentation completeness rates
- C. Audit a random sample of records for coding accuracy
- D. Calculate the average length of stay for each period

Answer: B — The most effective way to determine whether a CMI increase reflects a true change in patient acuity versus improved coding capture is to examine both the DRG distribution shift and documentation completeness metrics simultaneously. If higher-weighted DRGs are being assigned more frequently in the current period due to better documentation of complications and comorbidities (CCs and MCCs), that suggests a coding/documentation improvement. Comparing the MS-DRG distribution reveals which specific DRG pairs or families shifted; reviewing documentation completeness rates (such as query rates, CC/MCC capture rates, and physician response rates) identifies whether clinical documentation improvement activities drove the change. Recalculating CMI using only surgical DRGs (A) narrows the analysis to one service line and does not explain the overall shift; it would exclude medical DRGs where documentation improvement often has the greatest impact. Auditing a random sample for coding accuracy (C) is valuable for identifying errors but does not distinguish between acuity change and documentation improvement — both can produce accurate codes on audit. Average LOS (D) correlates with acuity and CMI, but an LOS change can lag CMI changes or be influenced by throughput factors independent of acuity.

16. A data integration team is designing an interface between a newly acquired community hospital's legacy ADT system and the health system's enterprise EHR. The legacy system uses a proprietary patient identifier format (six-digit numeric), while the enterprise system uses a 16-character alphanumeric medical record number. The team must ensure that the same patient is not registered as two separate records in the enterprise system. Which integration approach directly addresses this risk?

- A. HL7 FHIR bulk data export
- B. Enterprise master patient index (EMPI) with probabilistic matching
- C. Consolidation of source system databases into a single schema
- D. Implementation of a common data model

Answer: B — An enterprise master patient index (EMPI) is the standard solution for patient identity matching across systems with different identifier formats. An EMPI maintains a cross-reference of patient identifiers from all participating source systems and uses deterministic and/or probabilistic matching algorithms — comparing demographic attributes such as name, date of birth, address, and SSN — to link records belonging to the same individual across systems. This directly prevents duplicate patient registration. HL7 FHIR bulk data export (A) is a protocol for large-scale data retrieval from FHIR-compliant servers; it is a data exchange specification, not a patient identity management solution, and does not resolve identifier conflicts. Consolidating source system databases into a single schema (C) is a physical integration approach that would still require identity resolution logic before or during consolidation; without an EMPI, duplicate records would simply be merged into the same undifferentiated schema. A common data model (D) standardizes the structure and vocabulary of data for analytical purposes but operates downstream of patient registration and does not resolve real-time identity conflicts at the point of care.

17. A quality analyst is preparing a report on hospital-acquired condition (HAC) rates for the board of directors. She wants to display the HAC rate, the national benchmark, and the trend over 12 months in a single visualization that allows the board to quickly grasp performance status relative to goal. Which chart type is most appropriate?

- A. Box-and-whisker plot
- B. Combination line chart with reference line
- C. Treemap
- D. Funnel chart

Answer: B — A combination line chart with a reference line is the optimal choice for this reporting requirement. The monthly HAC rate can be plotted as a time-series line, the national benchmark displayed as a horizontal reference line, and the viewer can immediately assess whether performance is above or below the benchmark and identify the direction of the trend over 12 months. This single visualization answers all three of the analyst's stated needs. A box-and-whisker plot (A) displays the distribution of a variable — including quartiles and outliers — across categories; it does not effectively convey time-series trends or allow direct benchmark comparison in a board-level summary format. A treemap (C) uses nested rectangles to show hierarchical proportional data; it is designed for part-to-whole relationships across categories and is inappropriate for time-series performance tracking. A funnel chart (D) displays sequential stages in a process to show attrition or conversion rates; it has no application to tracking a rate metric against a benchmark over time.

18. A health information analyst is reviewing a patient's record and notices that the attending physician documented "respiratory failure" in the H&P but only "COPD exacerbation" in the discharge summary. The coding team is uncertain which condition to code. What should the coder do first, according to ICD-10-CM Official Guidelines?

- A. Code both conditions and let the claims adjudicator determine the principal diagnosis
- B. Query the attending physician to clarify whether respiratory failure was present on admission and whether it should be included in the final diagnosis
- C. Code only COPD exacerbation since the discharge summary supersedes all other documentation
- D. Code respiratory failure as an additional diagnosis because it is documented in the record

Answer: B — When documentation is conflicting or unclear between different parts of the medical record, the ICD-10-CM Official Guidelines direct the coding professional to query the physician for clarification rather than making an assumption. The discharge summary is the primary source for final diagnosis documentation, but contradictions between the H&P and discharge summary require clinical clarification — not a unilateral coding decision. The physician query process is the standard mechanism for resolving such ambiguity. Coding both conditions without clarification (A) risks submitting unsupported diagnosis codes; if respiratory failure was not clinically substantiated, coding it constitutes a compliance risk. The guideline that the discharge summary supersedes other documentation (C) applies to using it as the primary source, not as a blanket override of clinical contradictions that require physician input. Coding respiratory failure as an additional diagnosis based solely on H&P documentation (D) without physician confirmation that the condition was present and clinically significant is not appropriate when conflicting documentation exists.

19. A data warehouse architect is designing the schema for an analytics platform that must support complex queries across multiple years of inpatient, outpatient, and emergency department encounter data joined to laboratory and pharmacy records. Query performance is the primary concern; the platform will not be used for transactional processing. Which database schema design is most appropriate?

- A. Third normal form (3NF) relational schema
- B. Star schema with fact and dimension tables
- C. Object-oriented schema
- D. Fully denormalized flat file structure

Answer: B — A star schema organizes data around a central fact table (containing measurable events such as encounters) surrounded by dimension tables (patient, provider, facility, date, diagnosis, etc.). This design is optimized for analytical query performance because it minimizes the number of table joins required for complex aggregations, enables efficient columnar storage, and supports the type of multi-dimensional analysis described. Star schemas are the standard architecture for data warehouses and OLAP systems. A third normal form (3NF) schema (A) eliminates data redundancy and is appropriate for transactional (OLTP) systems where update integrity is critical; it requires many joins for analytical queries and degrades performance in reporting environments. An object-oriented schema (C) is designed for programming environments where data is stored as objects with methods; it is not standard practice for relational analytical databases. A fully denormalized flat file structure (D) eliminates all joins but creates massive data redundancy, storage inefficiency, and maintenance challenges that outweigh any query speed benefit; it is not a scalable or maintainable warehouse design for multi-year, multi-domain data.

20. A clinical data analyst is tasked with implementing a data quality monitoring program for the health system's medication reconciliation data. She wants to detect when the rate of incomplete medication reconciliations exceeds acceptable thresholds in near-real-time. Which data quality monitoring approach is most appropriate for an ongoing operational setting?

- A. Annual data quality audit with random sampling
- B. Retrospective benchmarking against industry standards
- C. Automated rules-based validation with alerting at the point of data entry or interface processing
- D. Periodic manual record review by pharmacy staff

Answer: C — Automated rules-based validation with alerting at the point of data entry or interface processing is the only approach among the options that provides near-real-time detection of data quality problems in an operational environment. By embedding validation rules in the EHR workflow or ETL process — such as flagging encounters where medication reconciliation is not completed within a defined window — the system can generate real-time alerts to clinical staff or supervisors, enabling immediate corrective action before the data quality problem compounds. An annual data quality audit with random sampling (A) is valuable for periodic assessment and compliance documentation but cannot detect or prevent near-real-time issues. Retrospective benchmarking against industry standards (B) compares aggregate performance after the fact; it is useful for strategic improvement planning but does not address near-real-time operational monitoring. Periodic manual record review by pharmacy staff (D) is labor-intensive, delayed, and subject to human error; it cannot scale to the volume of encounters in a health system and does not provide timely detection.

21. A health system is subject to a state law requiring it to submit patient-level discharge data to the state health department's all-payer claims database (APCD). A patient advocates that the hospital should not submit her data to the state because she has requested a restriction on certain disclosures under HIPAA. Under the interplay of HIPAA and state law, how should the hospital respond?

- A. Honor the patient's restriction request because HIPAA's right to restrict supersedes state reporting requirements
- B. Submit the data to the state because mandatory reporting to a public health authority is a permitted disclosure under HIPAA regardless of the patient's restriction request
- C. Submit only de-identified data to the state to balance compliance with the patient's request
- D. Seek an IRB waiver before submitting the data

Answer: B — HIPAA's Privacy Rule at 45 CFR §164.522(a) permits patients to request restrictions on certain uses and disclosures of their PHI, but covered entities are not required to agree to restriction requests, and even agreed-upon restrictions do not override legally mandated reporting obligations. Disclosures required by law — including mandatory state public health reporting and all-payer claims database submissions authorized under state statute — fall under permitted disclosures at 45 CFR §164.512 and are not subject to patient restriction requests. The hospital is legally required to comply with the state reporting mandate. Answer A is incorrect because HIPAA's restriction right does not override legally mandated disclosures — it applies to voluntary disclosures, not legally required ones. Answer C (submitting only de-identified data) is not permissible because state APCD statutes typically require patient-level data with sufficient identifiers to link records; unilaterally de-identifying would not satisfy the legal reporting obligation. Answer D (IRB waiver) applies to research disclosures, not mandatory public health reporting, and is not applicable here.

22. A hospital's revenue cycle department notices a significant increase in claim denials for a specific DRG over the past two quarters. The denials cite "not medically necessary — insufficient documentation." The HIM director launches a concurrent review process. Which intervention would most directly address the root cause of documentation-based medical necessity denials?

- A. Appeal all denied claims within 30 days
- B. Implement a clinical documentation improvement (CDI) program with concurrent physician query for high-denial DRGs
- C. Recode all affected claims to lower-weighted DRGs to avoid future denials
- D. Terminate the contracts with the payers issuing the denials

Answer: B — Medical necessity denials citing insufficient documentation indicate that the clinical record does not adequately capture the severity, complexity, or clinical rationale for the level of care billed. A clinical documentation improvement (CDI) program addresses the root cause by training physicians on documentation requirements for medical necessity, and by having CDI specialists conduct concurrent (real-time) record review and issue physician queries to prompt completion of documentation before claim submission. This directly reduces future denials by ensuring that the clinical record supports the assigned DRG at the time of coding. Appealing denied claims (A) is a reactive downstream process that recovers some revenue but does not prevent recurrence; it treats the symptom, not the cause. Recoding claims to lower-weighted DRGs (C) is not appropriate if the higher-weight DRG is clinically supported; it would reduce legitimate reimbursement and could misrepresent patient severity. Terminating payer contracts (D) is not a clinically or operationally viable response to documentation deficiencies and would harm patient access to care.

23. A data analyst is supporting a value-based care initiative and must calculate the risk-adjusted readmission rate for the health system. She applies a hierarchical logistic regression model that accounts for patient demographics, comorbidity burden, and social risk factors. After risk adjustment, the health system's observed-to-expected (O/E) readmission ratio is 0.88. How should this result be interpreted?

- A. The health system has 12% more readmissions than expected given its patient population
- B. The health system has 12% fewer readmissions than expected given its patient population, suggesting performance better than the risk-adjusted standard
- C. The risk adjustment model failed because the ratio should equal 1.0 for a well-calibrated model

- D. The 0.88 ratio indicates that 88% of expected readmissions were prevented

Answer: B — An observed-to-expected (O/E) ratio below 1.0 indicates that the observed number of readmissions is lower than the number predicted by the risk-adjustment model given the characteristics of the population served. An O/E of 0.88 means the health system had 12% fewer readmissions than expected for its patient mix, which is a favorable result suggesting performance better than the risk-adjusted benchmark. Answer A reverses the interpretation; a ratio greater than 1.0 (more observed than expected) would indicate excess readmissions. Answer C is incorrect because an O/E ratio of 1.0 would mean observed equals expected, not that the model is well-calibrated; model calibration is assessed by how accurately predicted probabilities match observed rates, not by whether the O/E ratio equals 1.0. Answer D is a misreading of the ratio as a percentage of prevented events; the 0.88 figure is a ratio of observed to expected counts, not a prevention rate.

24. A health information management analyst is asked to create a report on coding productivity for the inpatient coding team. She calculates that Coder A reviewed 18 records per day, Coder B reviewed 22 records per day, and Coder C reviewed 15 records per day over the same 30-day period. At the same time, quality audits reveal that Coder A had a 97% accuracy rate, Coder B had a 91% accuracy rate, and Coder C had a 99% accuracy rate. The coding manager wants to identify the coder with the best overall performance balancing productivity and quality. Which analytical approach best captures this combined performance?

- A. Rank coders by volume alone, since productivity is the primary measure for staffing decisions
- B. Calculate a composite score weighting accuracy more heavily than volume, since accuracy drives compliance and reimbursement integrity
- C. Report only accuracy rates to the compliance officer and only volume rates to the operations manager
- D. Calculate records per day only for records coded with 100% accuracy

Answer: B — Coding performance in a healthcare setting must balance productivity (throughput) and quality (accuracy), because errors in coding have direct consequences for reimbursement accuracy, compliance, and data integrity. A composite score that weights accuracy more heavily than volume reflects the regulatory and financial stakes: a coder who is fast but inaccurate creates compliance risk and reclassification liability. In this scenario, Coder B has the highest volume but the lowest accuracy; Coder C has the lowest volume but the highest accuracy; a weighted composite would allow the manager to evaluate the trade-off analytically. Ranking by volume alone (A) ignores accuracy and would falsely identify Coder B as the top performer despite the lowest accuracy rate. Splitting the report between two audiences (C) is a presentation choice, not an analytical approach, and prevents either stakeholder from understanding the performance trade-off. Calculating records per day only for perfect-accuracy records (D) creates a non-standard, artificially low productivity metric that does not reflect realistic operational performance and would penalize coders for any error, even minor ones.

25. A health system is preparing for an ONC Health IT Certification audit related to its EHR's 2015 Edition compliance. One of the required criteria involves patient electronic access to their health information. Under 21st Century Cures Act Final Rule requirements, what is the minimum standard the EHR must meet regarding patient access to their information via APIs?

- A. The EHR must provide patients with a PDF download of their complete medical record within 30 days of request
- B. The EHR must support a FHIR-based open API allowing patients to access their electronic health information (EHI) without special effort using third-party applications of their choice
- C. The EHR must provide read-only access to lab results and medications via a patient portal, with other record sections available by written request
- D. The EHR must encrypt all patient data transmissions but is not required to support third-party application access until 2030

Answer: B — The ONC 21st Century Cures Act Final Rule (85 FR 25642) requires certified health IT to support standardized, open FHIR APIs (HL7 FHIR Release 4 or later) enabling patients to access their electronic health information using applications of their choice without special effort. This includes the requirement for a SMART on FHIR-compliant patient-facing API that allows third-party apps to retrieve patient data with patient-authorized access. The rule specifically prohibits information blocking practices that would restrict this access. A PDF download within 30 days (A) may satisfy a HIPAA right-of-access request but does not meet the 21st Century Cures Act API requirement for electronic access via third-party applications. Read-only portal access limited to certain record sections (C) falls short of the full EHI access scope required by the rule and does not satisfy the open API requirement for third-party application access. The statement that open API requirements are deferred to 2030 (D) is factually incorrect; the ONC Final Rule implementation timelines for API access requirements were phased in beginning in 2022–2023, and no deferral to 2030 exists for this requirement.

.41 Questions 26–50

26. A regional health information exchange (HIE) wants to enable real-time clinical data sharing between a hospital EHR and a network of independent specialty clinics. The hospital system uses Epic and the clinics use a mix of athenahealth and eClinicalWorks. The HIE director asks you to recommend an interoperability standard that supports RESTful APIs, resource-based data models, and modern web protocols. Which standard best meets these requirements?

A. HL7 v2.5 messaging
B. CDA Release 2 with XDS.b transport
C. HL7 FHIR R4
D. ANSI X12 837 transaction set

Answer: C — FHIR R4 (Fast Healthcare Interoperability Resources) is specifically designed for RESTful API-based exchange using modern web protocols such as HTTP, JSON, and OAuth 2.0. It defines discrete resources (Patient, Observation, Encounter, etc.) that can be retrieved individually or in bundles, making it far more flexible than document-centric CDA or message-based HL7 v2. HL7 v2.5 is a legacy messaging standard that uses pipe-delimited segments and requires point-to-point interface engines, not RESTful APIs. CDA with XDS.b transport is document-oriented and does not natively support granular resource retrieval. ANSI X12 837 is a claims transaction standard for billing, not clinical interoperability.

27. A healthcare analytics team is designing a new enterprise data warehouse (EDW) to support reporting across inpatient, outpatient, and long-term care service lines. The data architect proposes organizing data into a central fact table for encounters with surrounding dimension tables for patient demographics, provider, facility, diagnosis, and time. What data warehouse design pattern is being described?

A. Third normal form (3NF) relational schema
B. Data vault modeling
C. Snowflake schema
D. Star schema

Answer: D — A star schema organizes a data warehouse with one central fact table containing measurable events (here, encounters with metrics such as LOS, charges, or visit counts) surrounded by denormalized dimension tables that describe the who, what, where, and when of those events. This design is optimized for analytical query performance and is the most common pattern in healthcare EDWs. A snowflake schema is related but normalizes the dimension tables into sub-dimensions, reducing redundancy at the cost of query complexity. Third normal form is appropriate for transactional OLTP systems but creates too many joins for analytical workloads. Data vault modeling uses hubs, links, and satellites and is optimized for auditability and incremental loading, not end-user reporting.

28. A population health team is conducting a community health needs assessment (CHNA) for a large urban hospital. The analyst pulls claims data showing elevated rates of emergency department visits for asthma among residents of three zip codes. The team wants to understand whether environmental, housing, or economic factors are driving these disparities. Which data source would best complement the claims data for this analysis?

A. Hospital discharge abstract data from the state all-payer claims database
B. HEDIS measure results from commercial payers
C. American Community Survey (ACS) data linked by census tract or zip code
D. CMS Hospital Compare publicly reported quality metrics

Answer: C — The American Community Survey (ACS) provides granular socioeconomic data including poverty rates, housing conditions, educational attainment, unemployment, and insurance coverage at the census tract or zip code level. Linking ACS data to claims data by geography allows the team to identify social determinants of health (SDOH) correlates of the asthma ED visit pattern. Hospital discharge data from an all-payer claims database would show the same utilization already captured in the claims extract and would not add SDOH context. HEDIS measures are plan-level quality metrics, not geographically granular SDOH data. CMS Hospital Compare reports facility-level quality measures and does not contain community-level demographic or economic information.

29. During an SDOH data integration project, a health system asks a data analyst to incorporate standardized social needs screening results from the EHR into the analytics data mart. The screening tool records responses using Z-code diagnoses from ICD-10-CM (e.g., Z59.0 for homelessness, Z63.0 for problems in relationship with spouse or partner). A governance committee asks how to ensure these codes are applied consistently across all outpatient clinics. Which approach best supports standardized SDOH documentation?

A. Allow each clinic to develop its own local coding guidelines for social needs
B. Implement a clinical decision support (CDSS) prompt tied to a standardized SDOH screening instrument that maps responses to the appropriate Z-codes
C. Require coders to assign Z-codes retrospectively by reviewing free-text nursing notes
D. Exclude Z-codes from the analytics data mart because they are not reimbursable diagnoses

Answer: B — Linking a standardized screening instrument (such as PRAPARE, AHC-HRSN, or Hunger Vital Sign) to a CDSS workflow that automatically maps positive responses to the corresponding Z-codes ensures consistent, complete, and structured SDOH documentation at the point of care. This approach reduces reliance on coder interpretation and minimizes documentation variability across sites. Allowing each clinic to develop its own guidelines creates inconsistency that undermines data comparability across the health system. Retrospective Z-code assignment from free-text notes is labor-intensive, error-prone, and subject to coder subjectivity. Excluding Z-codes because they are not reimbursable misunderstands their value for population health analytics, risk stratification, and federal quality reporting.

30. A large integrated delivery network (IDN) is preparing to incorporate patient-generated health data (PGHD) from consumer wearables—including step counts, heart rate, and sleep duration—into the clinical data repository for care management programs. The CHDA on the informatics team is asked to assess data quality before integration. Which data quality dimension is MOST at risk with wearable-sourced PGHD compared to EHR-sourced vitals?

A. Timeliness
B. Completeness
C. Accuracy and reliability
D. Consistency

Answer: C — Consumer-grade wearables are not FDA-cleared medical devices and their sensors introduce measurement variability, calibration drift, and algorithm-dependent interpretation (e.g., optical heart rate estimation). Accuracy and reliability are the primary data quality concerns because readings may systematically deviate from clinical-grade measurements. Timeliness is generally a strength of wearables, which produce continuous streams. Completeness may be an issue when patients stop wearing devices, but it is secondary to accuracy for clinical decision-making. Consistency across devices and platforms is a challenge but flows from the underlying accuracy problem rather than being an independent root cause.

31. A health system's data governance council is drafting a data stewardship policy for the enterprise analytics environment. The policy needs to assign accountability for data quality, metadata management, and access control decisions for each major data domain (clinical, financial, operational). Which governance role is BEST described as the individual who has business accountability for a specific data domain and the authority to approve access and define quality standards for that domain?

A. Data custodian
B. Data steward
C. Chief Data Officer
D. Database administrator

Answer: B — A data steward is a business-side subject matter expert who has been formally designated as accountable for the quality, definition, and appropriate use of data within a specific domain. The steward approves access requests, resolves data quality issues, maintains the data dictionary for their domain, and liaises with IT on implementation. A data custodian (often IT or database administration) is responsible for the technical storage, backup, and security controls but does not have business accountability for data content. The Chief Data Officer sets enterprise strategy and policy but does not manage day-to-day domain-level stewardship. The database administrator maintains the technical infrastructure and has no authority over data content policy.

32. An analyst working for a regional ACO is asked to evaluate the performance of the organization's diabetes management program. The analyst calculates the proportion of attributed patients with diabetes who had an HbA1c test in the past 12 months. This measure is reported as 74%. What type of quality measure is this, and which organization maintains the measure set most likely used to define it?

A. Outcome measure maintained by The Joint Commission (TJC)
B. Process measure maintained by NCQA through the HEDIS measure set
C. Structural measure maintained by CMS through the Physician Quality Reporting System
D. Efficiency measure maintained by the Agency for Healthcare Research and Quality (AHRQ)

Answer: B — The proportion of patients with diabetes who received an HbA1c test is a classic process measure—it captures whether a recommended clinical action was performed, not the result or outcome. NCQA's

HEDIS (Healthcare Effectiveness Data and Information Set) includes the Comprehensive Diabetes Care measure, which covers HbA1c testing frequency. HEDIS is the most widely used quality measure set in managed care and ACO settings. TJC measures focus on hospital accreditation and inpatient care processes. The Physician Quality Reporting System (PQRS) was a CMS program retired in 2016; its successor is the Merit-based Incentive Payment System (MIPS). Efficiency measures evaluate resource use relative to quality, which is not what the HbA1c testing rate represents.

33. A hospital CDI (clinical documentation improvement) department is analyzing physician query patterns. A data analyst discovers that 22% of cases coded as sepsis 3 (A41.9) lack documentation of a positive blood culture, a systemic inflammatory response, or an identified infectious source in the attending's notes. The CDI team wants to flag these cases prospectively before billing. Which tool or methodology is MOST appropriate for building this automated flagging logic?

A. Natural language processing (NLP) applied to clinical notes to detect absence of supporting documentation
B. ICD-10-CM Tabular List review
C. DRG grouper recalculation
D. Release of information (ROI) workflow audit

Answer: A — NLP can parse unstructured clinical notes to detect the presence or absence of clinical concepts such as documented infectious source, culture results, or SIRS criteria. Applying NLP prospectively to flag A41.9-coded cases lacking supporting documentation enables CDI specialists to query physicians before claims submission, reducing the risk of medical necessity denials or RAC audit findings. ICD-10-CM Tabular List review is a reference tool for coding guidance, not an automated flagging mechanism. DRG grouper recalculation validates that assigned codes produce the correct DRG weight but does not assess documentation adequacy. ROI workflow audits address disclosure processes, not CDI quality.

34. An epidemiologist at a state health department is studying the burden of opioid use disorder (OUD) in rural counties. She calculates that in County A, there are 142 new OUD diagnoses per 100,000 population in 2025. She compares this to County B, which has 89 new OUD diagnoses per 100,000 in the same period. Which epidemiological measure is she using, and what does it represent?

A. Prevalence — the total number of existing cases in a population at a given time
B. Incidence rate — the number of new cases arising in a defined population over a specified time period
C. Case fatality rate — the proportion of people with OUD who die from the disorder
D. Attack rate — the proportion of exposed individuals who develop the disease

Answer: B — The measure described is an incidence rate because it counts new diagnoses (new cases) arising in a defined population (county residents) over a defined time period (calendar year 2025), expressed per 100,000 population. Incidence measures disease onset and is used for monitoring trends and evaluating prevention interventions. Prevalence includes all existing cases (both new and ongoing) at a point in time or over a period, not just newly identified ones. Case fatality rate measures mortality among those already diagnosed and is not applicable here. Attack rate is used in outbreak investigations and represents the proportion of a specifically exposed group that develops disease.

35. A hospital quality department is building a dashboard for the hospital board of directors, most of whom are community business leaders and philanthropists without clinical backgrounds. The dashboard will report on three key quality indicators: 30-day readmission rate, hospital-acquired infection (HAI) rate, and patient satisfaction (HCAHPS). Which dashboard design principle is MOST important to apply for this audience?

A. Display raw numerator and denominator counts for each measure so board members can verify the calculations themselves
B. Use color-coded performance indicators (e.g., red/yellow/green) and plain-language labels that contextualize performance against national benchmarks
C. Present all measures in a single complex table with risk-adjustment methodology footnotes
D. Limit the dashboard to statistical process control (SPC) charts with upper and lower control limits

Answer: B — For a non-technical executive audience, effective dashboard design prioritizes immediate comprehension over analytical depth. Color-coded status indicators (traffic light formatting) allow board members to quickly identify areas of concern, while plain-language measure names and benchmark comparisons provide context without requiring statistical literacy. Raw numerator/denominator tables require the audience to calculate rates themselves and may obscure meaningful patterns. A single dense table with risk-adjustment footnotes overwhelms non-clinical readers and buries the story. SPC charts are powerful for operational quality improvement teams but require familiarity with statistical process control concepts that most board members do not have.

36. A CHDA is performing a gap analysis of a health system's data governance maturity. She discovers that the master patient index (MPI) contains approximately 8,400 duplicate patient records out of 620,000 total records—a 1.36% duplicate rate. These duplicates are causing patients to receive bills at wrong addresses and creating fragmented longitudinal records. Which capability is MOST essential to address this problem?

A. Implementing a new EHR system with a different database engine
B. Deploying probabilistic matching algorithms and an enterprise master patient index (EMPI) with merge/unmerge workflows
C. Requiring all patients to present two forms of government identification at registration
D. Purging all duplicate records from the database without review

Answer: B — Probabilistic matching algorithms score record pairs on multiple attributes (name, date of birth, address, SSN fragments, phone number) to identify likely duplicates even when fields have typographical errors or incomplete data. An enterprise MPI with merge and unmerge workflows allows trained staff to resolve potential duplicates with an auditable process and reverse errors. Implementing a new EHR does not resolve the existing duplicate records and may compound the problem during data migration. Requiring stricter patient identification at registration helps prevent future duplicates but does not resolve the existing 8,400. Purging records without review risks deleting legitimate patients and violates data retention regulations.

37. A health system data analyst is designing an ETL (extract, transform, load) process to populate a clinical data warehouse from five source systems: the EHR, the lab system, the pharmacy system, the radiology PACS, and the billing system. During the design phase, the analyst notes that the EHR assigns patients a medical record number (MRN), the billing system uses an account number, and the lab system uses a collection order ID. Which design decision MOST effectively resolves this patient identifier mismatch across source systems?

A. Use the billing account number as the universal patient key because it is present in all financial records
B. Generate a new surrogate key in the EDW that is linked to each source system's local identifier through a crosswalk table
C. Require each source system vendor to adopt the EHR's MRN before the ETL is built
D. Drop records from systems that do not share the EHR's MRN

Answer: B — Creating a surrogate key (a system-generated integer or UUID) in the EDW and maintaining a crosswalk table that maps each source system's local identifier (MRN, account number, order ID) to the surrogate key is the standard data warehousing solution for cross-system patient identity. This approach is vendor-agnostic, preserves source identifiers for lineage tracing, and accommodates new source systems without redesigning the schema. Using the billing account number as a universal key fails because one patient may have multiple account numbers and the lab and radiology systems may not use it at all. Requiring all vendors to adopt the EHR MRN is operationally impractical and may take years. Dropping records from non-MRN systems creates catastrophic gaps in the longitudinal patient record.

38. An accountable care organization (ACO) is performing risk stratification to identify high-need patients for a new complex care management program. The analytics team is considering three approaches: (1) using HCC (Hierarchical Condition Category) risk scores derived from claims, (2) using a predictive model trained on EHR data to predict 12-month hospitalization probability, and (3) using a composite score combining claims-based HCC scores, prior ED utilization, and a social needs screening result. A governance committee asks which approach best supports both clinical prioritization and equitable patient selection. Which approach is MOST defensible?

A. Approach 1 only — HCC scores are the CMS-validated standard for risk adjustment
B. Approach 2 only — machine learning models are more accurate than administrative claims
C. Approach 3 — a composite score that integrates clinical risk, utilization patterns, and SDOH produces a more complete and equitable picture of patient need
D. None of the above — risk stratification should rely solely on physician judgment

Answer: C — Combining claims-based risk scores (HCC), utilization history (ED frequency), and social needs data into a composite risk score captures multiple dimensions of vulnerability that no single data source reflects adequately. HCC scores alone measure diagnosis-based clinical complexity but miss unmet social needs and acute utilization behavior. Predictive models trained on EHR data can embed historical care inequities into their predictions, perpetuating disparate access to care management. Composite approaches allow the organization to intentionally weight social risk factors, which is increasingly required by CMS innovation models and equity frameworks. Physician judgment alone is unscalable and subject to implicit bias without systematic data support.

39. A CHDA is evaluating a vendor's proposal to implement a natural language processing (NLP) tool that will extract problem list diagnoses from unstructured clinical notes for population health reporting. The vendor claims the tool has a sensitivity of 91% and a specificity of 88% for detecting diabetes diagnoses in physician notes. How should the CHDA interpret these statistics when advising the governance committee?

A. A sensitivity of 91% means the tool will correctly identify 91% of patients who have a diabetes diagnosis documented in their notes; a specificity of 88% means 12% of patients without diabetes will be incorrectly flagged as having it
B. A sensitivity of 91% means 91% of all notes processed will be returned without errors; specificity of 88% means 88% of extracted terms will match the ICD-10-CM code set
C. Both sensitivity and specificity above 90% guarantee that the tool is ready for production use without further validation
D. Sensitivity and specificity are not meaningful metrics for NLP evaluation; only F1 score should be considered

Answer: A — Sensitivity (recall) measures the tool's ability to correctly identify true positive cases—here, the 91% of patients with documented diabetes that the NLP correctly captures. Specificity measures the tool's ability to correctly identify true negatives—patients without diabetes who are correctly excluded; 88% specificity means 12% of those without the diagnosis will be falsely flagged (false positive rate). These two values reflect a trade-off: high sensitivity reduces missed diagnoses at the cost of more false positives. The governance committee must decide whether the false positive rate is acceptable for downstream reporting uses. The 91%/88% figures apply to the validation dataset and do not guarantee production readiness without site-specific validation on the health system's own notes.

40. A hospital is preparing to submit an electronic clinical quality measure (eCQM) to CMS for the Hospital Inpatient Quality Reporting (IQR) program. The measure requires data elements from both structured EHR data and claims. The analyst needs to understand the file format CMS requires for eCQM submission. Which file format is used for CMS eCQM submissions?

A. HL7 FHIR R4 Bundle in NDJSON format
B. QRDA Category I (patient-level) or QRDA Category III (aggregate) XML documents
C. CDA Consolidated Clinical Document Release 2 (C-CDA)
D. ANSI X12 837P professional claim transactions

Answer: B — CMS accepts eCQM data in Quality Reporting Document Architecture (QRDA) format. QRDA Category I is a patient-level XML document containing individual patient data used to calculate measure performance. QRDA Category III is an aggregate XML document that reports measure results across a population. Both are HL7-defined standards specifically designed for clinical quality measure reporting to CMS programs including IQR, MIPS, and Medicaid quality initiatives. FHIR R4 NDJSON bundles are used for Bulk Data Access and some newer CMS interoperability rules but are not the current submission format for IQR eCQMs. C-CDA is a clinical document standard for care transitions and referrals, not quality measure reporting. The 837P is a billing transaction, not a quality reporting format.

41. An analyst at a Medicaid managed care organization is building a report on inpatient utilization for attributed members. She pulls data and finds that 3,200 admissions are associated with 2,800 unique members over a 12-month period. She wants to calculate the admission rate per 1,000 member months. The plan has 85,000 member months for the period. What is the correct rate?

A. 3,200 ÷ 85,000 × 1,000 = 37.6 admissions per 1,000 member months
B. 2,800 ÷ 85,000 × 1,000 = 32.9 admissions per 1,000 member months
C. 3,200 ÷ 2,800 × 1,000 = 1,142.9 admissions per 1,000 members
D. 2,800 ÷ 3,200 × 1,000 = 875 members per 1,000 admissions

Answer: A — The inpatient admission rate per 1,000 member months is calculated by dividing the total number of admissions (3,200) by the total member months (85,000) and multiplying by 1,000. This yields 37.6 admissions per 1,000 member months. Member months (not unique members) is the correct denominator because it accounts for variable enrollment durations across the reporting period—members who were enrolled for only part of the year contribute proportionally to the denominator. Using unique members (2,800) as the denominator would undercount enrollment time and produce an inflated rate. Options C and D compute ratios that are not standard utilization metrics.

42. A health system data governance team is reviewing its de-identification policy in preparation for a research data sharing agreement. The team wants to ensure the dataset meets HIPAA Safe Harbor de-identification standards. A researcher asks whether the dataset can include the patient's five-digit zip code. What is the correct guidance under HIPAA Safe Harbor?

A. Five-digit zip codes are permitted under Safe Harbor if the dataset has fewer than 500 patients
B. Five-digit zip codes must be removed or generalized to the first three digits, and only if the three-digit zip

code covers more than 20,000 people
C. Five-digit zip codes are always prohibited under Safe Harbor regardless of population size
D. Five-digit zip codes are permitted as long as the researcher signs a data use agreement (DUA)

Answer: B — Under HIPAA Safe Harbor (45 CFR §164.514(b)), the geographic standard is that zip codes must be generalized to the first three digits, and even three-digit codes must be suppressed (replaced with "000") if the geographic unit contains 20,000 or fewer people according to current Census data. If the three-digit prefix covers more than 20,000 people, it may be retained. Five-digit zip codes are always prohibited under Safe Harbor because they can identify individuals in small communities. The size of the dataset (500 patients) is irrelevant to the zip code rule. A data use agreement does not authorize the retention of Safe Harbor-prohibited identifiers.

43. A hospital compliance department is investigating a potential HIPAA breach involving access to patient records in the EHR. The audit log shows that a nurse practitioner accessed 340 patient records over a 30-day period without a documented clinical relationship to those patients. What is the appropriate HIPAA term for accessing PHI without a permissible purpose, and what professional ethics principle does this violate most directly?

A. Incidental disclosure; beneficence
B. Minimum necessary standard violation; non-maleficence
C. Unauthorized access (snooping); patient privacy and confidentiality
D. Treatment exception; justice

Answer: C — Accessing patient records without a clinical or operational need is commonly called "snooping" and constitutes an unauthorized use or disclosure of protected health information (PHI) under HIPAA. It violates the core health information management (HIM) ethics principle of patient privacy and confidentiality—the obligation to access and use PHI only for legitimate, authorized purposes. Incidental disclosure refers to unavoidable secondary exposures during otherwise permissible activities, which does not apply here. The minimum necessary standard requires limiting PHI access to what is needed for a specific purpose, and while it is relevant, the primary characterization is unauthorized access. The treatment exception permits access by providers involved in a patient's care; it does not apply to providers with no clinical relationship.

44. A population health analyst is tasked with evaluating the effectiveness of a diabetes prevention program (DPP) offered by a health system. The program enrolled 450 pre-diabetic patients over 18 months. The analyst wants to compare diabetes onset rates between program participants and non-participants while controlling for baseline characteristics such as age, BMI, HbA1c at baseline, and insurance type. Which analytical approach is MOST appropriate?

A. Descriptive frequency tables comparing participant demographics to the general population
B. Matched cohort analysis or multivariable logistic regression adjusting for baseline confounders
C. A simple pre/post comparison of HbA1c values within the enrolled group only
D. A cross-sectional prevalence comparison between zip codes with and without program sites

Answer: B — Because DPP enrollment was not randomized, participants likely differ systematically from non-participants (e.g., higher health literacy, more engaged with the health system). Matched cohort analysis pairs each participant with a comparable non-participant on key confounders, or multivariable logistic regression statistically adjusts for those confounders, allowing a more valid estimate of program effect. Frequency tables are descriptive and do not support causal inference. A pre/post comparison within the enrolled group only has no control group and cannot distinguish program effects from natural disease progression or regression to the mean. Cross-sectional zip code comparisons introduce ecological fallacy and do not control for individual-level confounders.

45. A data analyst is reviewing a hospital's data dictionary and notices that the field "discharge_disposition" has 14 distinct values in the production database but only 12 values are documented in the data dictionary, and two values are not defined anywhere. Which data governance process should be initiated to resolve this discrepancy?

A. Delete the two undocumented values from the database immediately to restore consistency
B. Initiate a data quality incident with the domain data steward to investigate the source and meaning of the undocumented values and update the data dictionary accordingly
C. Map the two undocumented values to the closest existing defined values without investigation
D. Issue a corrective action to the EHR vendor for creating undocumented codes

Answer: B — A discrepancy between the data dictionary and the production database is a data quality incident that requires investigation by the domain data steward, who has the business authority to determine whether the undocumented values represent new legitimate dispositions (e.g., added by a vendor update), data entry errors, or legacy codes that were never retired. The data dictionary must be updated to reflect the authoritative definition. Deleting database values without investigation risks destroying valid clinical or financial information. Mapping without investigation may misclassify patients and corrupt downstream reports. Issuing a vendor corrective action may eventually be warranted but is premature before the root cause is established.

46. An HIE is implementing TEFCA (Trusted Exchange Framework and Common Agreement) to enable nationwide health information exchange. A CHDA is asked to explain the role of a Qualified Health Information Network (QHIN) in the TEFCA framework. Which statement BEST describes a QHIN's function?

A. A QHIN is a government agency that certifies EHR systems for meaningful use compliance
B. A QHIN is a network operator that signs the Common Agreement with ONC and serves as an interoperability intermediary enabling exchange among its participants and with other QHINs
C. A QHIN is a patient advocacy organization that manages consent preferences for nationwide data sharing
D. A QHIN is a cloud storage provider that hosts PHI on behalf of healthcare organizations under a BAA

Answer: B — Under TEFCA, Qualified Health Information Networks are entities (typically existing HIEs, networks, or health IT organizations) that agree to ONC's Common Agreement and serve as the technical and governance backbone for exchange. QHINs connect their participant organizations (providers, payers, PHAs) and route queries and responses between networks, enabling a nationwide network of networks. ONC designates QHINs through its recognized coordinating entity; as of 2025, the RCE is The Sequoia Project. QHINs are not government agencies, patient advocacy groups, or cloud storage providers—they are network operators with defined exchange obligations under the Common Agreement.

47. A CHDA is advising a hospital finance team on calculating the days not final billed (DNFB) metric for the inpatient coding department. The team asks what the DNFB metric measures and what its significance is. Which answer is MOST accurate?

A. DNFB measures the total number of inpatient accounts that have been coded but not yet submitted to payers, expressed in days of average revenue
B. DNFB measures the number of days between patient discharge and the assignment of the final ICD-10-CM/PCS codes and DRG, used to identify coding backlog
C. DNFB represents the total dollar value of inpatient accounts with discharged but not final billed status, expressed as days of average daily revenue, and serves as a key indicator of revenue cycle efficiency and cash flow risk
D. DNFB is the number of calendar days a payer has to remit payment after receiving a clean claim under contractual terms

Answer: C — Days Not Final Billed (DNFB) is a revenue cycle metric that quantifies the total charges held in accounts where patients have been discharged but claims have not yet been submitted, expressed as the equivalent number of days of average daily net revenue. It reflects a combination of unbilled accounts due to coding delays, clinical documentation holds, charge capture issues, and compliance review holds. High DNFB indicates cash flow risk and operational inefficiency. Option B describes the coding lag (discharge-to-final-code interval), which is a component of DNFB but not the complete metric. Option A describes only coded-not-billed accounts, which is one category within DNFB. Option D describes the contractual payment terms (timely filing) between provider and payer.

48. A regional health system is building a population health analytics platform and wants to incorporate FHIR Bulk Data Access to retrieve large volumes of patient data from its EHR for a payer-provider data exchange. The technical team asks the CHDA to explain what NDJSON format means in this context and why it is used. Which explanation is correct?

A. NDJSON (Newline-Delimited JSON) is a format in which each line of a file contains a complete, valid JSON object representing a single FHIR resource, enabling efficient streaming and parallel processing of large datasets
B. NDJSON is a compressed binary format used by FHIR servers to encrypt PHI during bulk data transfer
C. NDJSON is a proprietary Microsoft format that requires Azure cloud infrastructure to parse
D. NDJSON is an XML schema standard used by ONC to define the USCDI data elements required under the 21st Century Cures Act

Answer: A — NDJSON (Newline-Delimited JSON, also called JSON Lines) is the file format specified by the HL7 FHIR Bulk Data Access Implementation Guide for asynchronous export of large FHIR datasets. Each line in an NDJSON file is a self-contained JSON object representing one FHIR resource (e.g., one Patient resource, one Observation). This line-by-line structure enables streaming parsers to process files without loading the entire dataset into memory, and supports parallel processing by splitting files at newline boundaries. NDJSON is not binary, not encrypted, not Microsoft-proprietary, and not an XML standard—it is a plain-text format widely supported by open-source tools.

49. A CHDA at a quality improvement organization is reviewing a hospital's performance on the CMS Excess Days in Acute Care (EDAC) measure for heart failure patients. The measure penalizes hospitals for patients who have unplanned ED visits, observation stays, or readmissions within 30 days of discharge. The analyst finds that the hospital's EDAC ratio is 1.18, meaning it has 18% more excess days than the national mean. The quality team asks what this means for the hospital's value-based purchasing (VBP) penalties. Which statement is MOST accurate?

A. An EDAC ratio above 1.0 means the hospital's performance is better than expected and will result in a VBP bonus
B. An EDAC ratio of 1.18 means the hospital has 18% more acute care utilization post-discharge than the risk-adjusted national mean, which contributes to penalties under the Hospital Readmissions Reduction Program (HRRP)
C. EDAC ratios above 1.0 trigger automatic termination from the Medicare program
D. The EDAC ratio is only reported publicly and has no connection to Medicare payment adjustments

Answer: B — An EDAC ratio greater than 1.0 indicates that the hospital's post-discharge acute care utilization exceeds what is expected given its patient case mix, meaning it performs worse than the national benchmark. While EDAC is a distinct measure from the Hospital Readmissions Reduction Program (HRRP), high EDAC performance signals inadequate post-discharge care transitions and often correlates with HRRP penalties, which reduce Medicare base operating DRG payments by up to 3% for excess readmissions in heart failure, AMI, COPD, pneumonia, CABG, and hip/knee replacement. An EDAC ratio above 1.0 is not a bonus indicator, does not trigger program termination, and is not reporting-only—it directly informs CMS payment policy analysis.

50. A CHDA is facilitating a PDSA (Plan-Do-Study-Act) cycle to improve the accuracy of problem list documentation in a large multispecialty outpatient practice. In the "Study" phase, the team reviews data collected during a six-week pilot in which a CDSS prompt reminded physicians to reconcile problem lists at the time of visit documentation. The team finds that problem list accuracy improved from 61% to 74% during the pilot but also that physician satisfaction with the CDSS prompt declined by 22 percentage points. What is the MOST appropriate action in the "Act" phase based on these findings?

A. Abandon the intervention because physician satisfaction declined
B. Immediately scale the intervention to all 48 practice sites without modification
C. Modify the intervention—such as adjusting prompt timing, frequency, or design—to preserve the accuracy gains while reducing alert fatigue, then plan a new PDSA cycle to test the revised approach
D. Conclude that a 13-percentage-point improvement is insufficient and discard all data

Answer: C — The PDSA cycle is an iterative quality improvement methodology. The "Act" phase requires the team to decide whether to adopt, adapt, or abandon the intervention based on evidence from the Study phase. The data present a mixed result: clinical quality improved meaningfully (13 percentage points) but provider satisfaction declined substantially, signaling alert fatigue risk that could undermine sustainability. The appropriate Act response is to adapt—redesign the prompt to be less intrusive (e.g., ambient suggestion vs. interruptive alert, fewer trigger conditions, or batched reminders) while retaining the reconciliation workflow. A new PDSA cycle then tests the refined intervention. Abandoning the intervention ignores a meaningful clinical improvement. Scaling immediately without modification spreads the physician satisfaction problem across the enterprise. Discarding data based on a predetermined improvement threshold is not consistent with evidence-based QI methodology.

.42 Glossary of Key Terms

ACO (Accountable Care Organization) — A group of doctors, hospitals, and other healthcare providers who voluntarily coordinate care for Medicare and commercially insured patients to deliver high-quality, cost-efficient care. ACOs share savings when they hit quality benchmarks while keeping spending below a benchmark, and may share losses in two-sided risk models.

ADT (Admission, Discharge, Transfer) — A category of HL7 messages (A01, A02, A03, etc.) generated by hospital registration and patient tracking systems to notify downstream systems and care team members of changes in patient location, status, or care setting. ADT feeds are foundational data sources for HIEs and real-time analytics platforms.

AHC-HRSN (Accountable Health Communities Health-Related Social Needs) — A standardized 10-question screening instrument developed through the CMS Accountable Health Communities model to assess patients' social needs across five core domains: housing instability, food insecurity, transportation problems, utility help needs, and interpersonal safety. Designed to map to Z-code diagnoses in ICD-10-CM.

API (Application Programming Interface) — A defined set of protocols, endpoints, and data formats that allow software applications to communicate with one another programmatically. In health IT, RESTful APIs using FHIR resources are the emerging standard for EHR data access under ONC's 21st Century Cures Act rules.

Attribution — The process of assigning patients to a specific provider, practice, or payer for the purpose of quality reporting, performance measurement, or value-based payment. Attribution algorithms use claims, enrollment, or EHR data and may be prospective (predictive) or retrospective (based on historical care patterns).

Benchmark — A standard or reference point used to evaluate performance. In healthcare analytics, benchmarks may be national (e.g., HEDIS national percentiles), regional (e.g., state Medicaid mean), or internal (e.g., prior-year performance). Benchmarks provide context that transforms a raw rate into actionable performance information.

BI (Business Intelligence) — A set of technologies, tools, and practices for collecting, integrating, analyzing, and presenting enterprise data to support decision-making. BI platforms (such as Tableau, Power BI, and Qlik) provide dashboards, reports, and self-service analytics capabilities for operational, financial, and clinical data.

C-CDA (Consolidated Clinical Document Architecture) — An HL7 standard for clinical document templates that defines structured XML documents for common care transitions and clinical summaries, including Continuity of Care Documents (CCD), Discharge Summaries, Progress Notes, and Referral Notes. C-CDA is mandated by ONC certification criteria for EHR interoperability.

Cardinality — In database design, the number of distinct values in a column or the numerical relationship between rows in related tables (one-to-one, one-to-many, many-to-many). High cardinality means many unique values (e.g., patient ID); low cardinality means few distinct values (e.g., sex, Y/N flags). Cardinality informs indexing strategy and dimension table design.

Case Mix Index (CMI) — The average relative weight of all Medicare inpatient cases discharged from a hospital, calculated by summing all MS-DRG weights and dividing by the total number of cases. A higher CMI reflects a more clinically complex patient population and is associated with higher resource consumption and reimbursement.

CDI (Clinical Documentation Improvement) — A program within health information management that focuses on ensuring physician documentation in the medical record fully and accurately reflects the patient's clinical status, supporting accurate coding, appropriate DRG assignment, quality measure reporting, and risk adjustment. CDI specialists review records and query physicians for clarifying documentation.

CDSS (Clinical Decision Support System) — Software that provides clinicians with patient-specific assessments or recommendations derived from clinical knowledge bases, evidence-based guidelines, and patient data. Examples include drug-allergy alerts, best practice advisories, order sets, and diagnostic support. CDSS is embedded in EHRs and can be rule-based or machine learning-driven.

Claim — A formal request submitted by a provider to a payer for reimbursement for services rendered to a patient. Claims contain administrative, demographic, and clinical data elements (diagnosis codes, procedure codes, revenue codes, charges) formatted to ANSI X12 or CMS-1500/UB-04 standards.

Clean Claim — A claim that passes all payer edits and contains all required information for adjudication without requiring additional information or correction. Clean claims are processed within defined timely payment windows under state prompt payment laws; denial rates and clean claim rates are key revenue cycle performance indicators.

CMS (Centers for Medicare & Medicaid Services) — The federal agency within the U.S. Department of Health and Human Services that administers Medicare, Medicaid, the Children's Health Insurance Program (CHIP), and the ACA marketplace. CMS sets coverage, payment, and quality reporting policies that drive most healthcare data and analytics requirements.

Cohort — A defined group of patients who share one or more characteristics (e.g., a diagnosis, a procedure, an enrollment date, an exposure) and who are followed over time for analytical or research purposes. Cohort studies compare outcomes between exposed and unexposed groups to estimate associations or intervention effects.

Confounding Variable — A variable that is associated with both the exposure of interest and the outcome, creating a spurious or distorted association between them. For example, age may confound the relationship between a treatment and mortality if older patients are both more likely to receive the treatment and more likely to die. Confounders must be controlled through study design or statistical adjustment.

CQL (Clinical Quality Language) — A Health Level Seven (HL7) standard authoring language used to express the logic for electronic clinical quality measures (eCQMs) and clinical decision support rules in a computable, human-readable format. CQL is used in conjunction with FHIR-based quality measure frameworks and QRDA submission specifications.

CRISP-DM (Cross-Industry Standard Process for Data Mining) — A widely used six-phase framework for data science and analytics projects: Business Understanding, Data Understanding, Data Preparation, Modeling, Evaluation, and Deployment. CRISP-DM provides a structured methodology that is vendor-neutral and applicable to healthcare analytics projects from predictive modeling to NLP development.

Data Dictionary — A centralized repository that defines and describes all data elements in a database or information system, including field names, data types, permissible values, definitions, business rules, and source system mappings. A well-maintained data dictionary is foundational to data governance, enabling consistent interpretation of data across the organization.

Data Element — The smallest named unit of data that has meaning in a specific context—a single attribute or field, such as "date_of_birth," "primary_diagnosis_code," or "length_of_stay." Data elements are defined in data dictionaries and data standards such as USCDI. In FHIR, data elements are mapped to specific resource attributes.

Data Lake — A centralized storage repository that holds large volumes of raw, unstructured, semi-structured, and structured data in its native format until it is needed for analysis. Unlike a data warehouse, a data lake does not impose a schema at ingestion; schema is applied at read time ("schema-on-read"). Data lakes are common in cloud-based healthcare analytics architectures.

Data Lineage — The documentation of data's origins, the transformations it has undergone, and the path it has traveled from source system to final use. Data lineage enables analysts to trace an analytic result back to its source, identify where errors were introduced, and demonstrate compliance with data governance policies.

Data Mart — A subset of a data warehouse that is focused on a specific subject area, department, or business function (e.g., a cardiology outcomes data mart, a revenue cycle data mart). Data marts are tailored for the analytical needs of a specific user group and typically draw from the enterprise data warehouse.

Data Quality Dimensions — The attributes used to assess whether data is fit for its intended use. Widely recognized dimensions include accuracy (correctness), completeness (no missing values), timeliness (currency), consistency (agreement across sources), validity (conformance to defined formats or value sets), and uniqueness (absence of duplicates). AHIMA and AHIMA's data quality framework define these as core governance concepts.

Data Steward — A business-side subject matter expert who is formally accountable for the quality, definitions, and appropriate use of data within a specific domain. Data stewards approve data access, resolve quality issues, maintain the data dictionary, and serve as the liaison between business users and the technical data management team.

De-identification — The process of removing or obscuring protected health information (PHI) from a dataset so that the remaining information cannot reasonably identify an individual. HIPAA provides two methods: Safe Harbor (removing 18 specified identifier categories) and Expert Determination (statistical and scientific certification that re-identification risk is very small).

DNFB (Days Not Final Billed) — A revenue cycle metric that quantifies the value of discharged inpatient accounts that have not yet been submitted to payers, expressed as the equivalent number of days of average daily net revenue. DNFB reflects combined delays from coding, documentation, charge capture, and compliance holds and is a key indicator of cash flow risk.

DRG (Diagnosis-Related Group) — A patient classification system used by Medicare and other payers to set prospective payment rates for inpatient hospital stays. Each DRG represents a group of clinically similar diagnoses or procedures with similar expected resource consumption. MS-DRG (Medicare Severity DRG) is the current CMS grouping system, with over 760 groups stratified by complication and comorbidity level.

eCQM (Electronic Clinical Quality Measure) — A quality measure that uses data from electronic health records and other health IT systems to assess the quality of care provided. eCQMs are defined using standardized logic (CQL) and submitted to CMS in QRDA format. They replace paper-based chart-abstracted measures in federal quality reporting programs.

EDW (Enterprise Data Warehouse) — A centralized analytical database that integrates data from multiple operational source systems across an organization. Unlike transactional databases, an EDW is optimized for complex queries, aggregations, and historical trend analysis. In healthcare, EDWs typically integrate EHR, claims, billing, and operational data.

EHR (Electronic Health Record) — A digital version of a patient's medical history that is created and maintained by a provider organization. Certified EHRs must meet ONC health IT certification criteria and support structured data capture, clinical decision support, and interoperability. EHRs are the primary source system for most healthcare analytics work.

ETL (Extract, Transform, Load) — The data integration process of extracting data from source systems, transforming it to conform to the target schema and data quality standards (cleaning, mapping, aggregating), and loading it into a destination system such as a data warehouse or data mart. ETL pipelines are the backbone of healthcare EDW population.

FHIR (Fast Healthcare Interoperability Resources) — An HL7 standard for health data exchange that uses modern web technologies (RESTful APIs, JSON/XML, OAuth 2.0). FHIR defines over 140 discrete resources representing clinical and administrative data elements. FHIR R4 is the current mandated version for ONC certification under the 21st Century Cures Act.

Gap Analysis — A systematic comparison of current performance or capabilities against a desired standard, target, or best practice to identify areas requiring improvement. In healthcare analytics, gap analysis is used in data governance maturity assessments, quality measure performance reviews, and IT capability planning.

HEDIS (Healthcare Effectiveness Data and Information Set) — A set of standardized performance measures developed and maintained by NCQA to assess health plan quality across domains including preventive care, chronic disease management, behavioral health, and access to care. Over 90% of U.S. health plans report HEDIS measures, making it the most widely used quality measurement tool in managed care.

HCC (Hierarchical Condition Category) — A risk adjustment model used by CMS to predict the expected healthcare costs of Medicare Advantage enrollees based on their demographic characteristics and diagnosis history from claims. HCC scores are used to set capitated payment rates and risk-stratify patients for care management programs.

HIE (Health Information Exchange) — The electronic sharing of clinical information across organizational boundaries to support patient care, public health, and analytics. HIEs may operate as query-based (pull), directed (push/secure messaging), or consumer-mediated networks. TEFCA is the federal framework for establishing a nationwide HIE infrastructure.

HIPAA (Health Insurance Portability and Accountability Act) — Federal legislation enacted in 1996 that establishes national standards for the protection of individually identifiable health information (protected health information, or PHI), electronic health information security, and administrative simplification of healthcare transactions. The HIPAA Privacy Rule, Security Rule, Breach Notification Rule, and Omnibus Rule are implemented by OCR within HHS.

HL7 (Health Level Seven International) — A global standards development organization that creates standards for the exchange, integration, sharing, and retrieval of electronic health information. HL7 standards include HL7 v2 messaging, CDA, FHIR, CQL, and QRDA. "Level seven" refers to the application layer of the OSI model.

HIM (Health Information Management) — A profession focused on the acquisition, analysis, and protection of digital and traditional medical information required to provide healthcare. HIM professionals manage medical records, coding, release of information, data quality, and increasingly analytics and informatics functions. AHIMA is the primary professional association.

Informatics — The science of information management, including how data is collected, organized, analyzed, and used to support decisions. Health informatics encompasses clinical informatics, nursing informatics, public health informatics, and consumer health informatics. CHDA candidates draw on informatics principles for data system design and analytical methodology.

ICD-10-CM (International Classification of Diseases, 10th Revision, Clinical Modification) — The U.S. clinical modification of WHO's ICD-10 classification system, used to code diagnoses, symptoms, and reasons for encounters in all U.S. healthcare settings. ICD-10-CM contains over 70,000 codes and is maintained jointly by CDC and NCHS. It replaced ICD-9-CM on October 1, 2015.

ICD-10-PCS (International Classification of Diseases, 10th Revision, Procedure Coding System) — The U.S. system for coding inpatient hospital procedures, used only in acute care settings for facility billing and data reporting. ICD-10-PCS contains over 87,000 alphanumeric codes with a seven-character structure. It replaced ICD-9-CM Volume 3 and is maintained by CMS.

Information Governance (IG) — An organizationwide framework of policies, accountabilities, and processes that ensure the availability, usability, integrity, and security of information. AHIMA defines IG as a set of multi-disciplinary structures that address the full lifecycle of organizational information to meet operational and strategic objectives. IG is broader than data governance and encompasses regulatory compliance, legal hold, and risk management.

IRB (Institutional Review Board) — A formally designated committee that reviews research involving human subjects to ensure ethical conduct, including protection of participants' rights, privacy, and welfare. IRBs apply federal regulations (45 CFR Part 46, Common Rule) and must approve or exempt studies before data collection begins. Use of patient data for research typically requires IRB review.

KPI (Key Performance Indicator) — A quantifiable metric used to evaluate the degree to which an organization, team, or process is achieving key objectives. In healthcare analytics, KPIs may include readmission rates, DNFB days, patient satisfaction scores, HEDIS measure rates, and cost per episode of care. Effective KPIs are specific, measurable, actionable, relevant, and time-bound (SMART).

Limited Data Set — Under HIPAA, a partially de-identified dataset from which certain direct identifiers (names, addresses, phone numbers, SSNs) have been removed, but which may still contain dates (including birth dates, admission dates) and geographic data at the city, state, or zip code level. A limited data set may be disclosed for research, public health, or healthcare operations under a data use agreement (DUA) without individual patient authorization.

Longitudinal Record — A comprehensive record of a patient's health history across time, providers, and care settings. A longitudinal record integrates data from multiple encounters and organizations to present a continuous view of the patient's diagnoses, medications, procedures, and results. Longitudinal records are essential for population health management and care coordination.

MPI (Master Patient Index) — A database that maintains a unique identifier for each patient served by a healthcare organization or network, along with key demographic attributes used for patient matching. The MPI is the foundation of the longitudinal patient record and is critical for data quality; duplicate records in the MPI cause fragmented care histories and billing errors.

NCQA (National Committee for Quality Assurance) — A private, nonprofit organization that develops and administers accreditation standards and quality measures for health plans, medical groups, and other healthcare organizations. NCQA is best known for HEDIS (Healthcare Effectiveness Data and Information Set) and Patient-Centered Medical Home (PCMH) recognition programs.

NDJSON (Newline-Delimited JSON) — A file format in which each line of a text file contains a complete, valid JSON object, allowing large datasets to be streamed and processed line by line without loading the entire file into memory. NDJSON is the required format for FHIR Bulk Data Access (export) operations, where each file contains all resources of a single resource type.

NLP (Natural Language Processing) — A branch of artificial intelligence that enables computers to understand, interpret, and generate human language text. In healthcare analytics, NLP is applied to extract structured clinical concepts (diagnoses, medications, procedures, social needs) from unstructured physician notes, radiology reports, discharge summaries, and patient-generated text.

ONC (Office of the National Coordinator for Health Information Technology) — The principal federal entity within HHS that coordinates national health IT policy, standards, and programs. ONC administers the EHR certification program under HITECH, develops USCDI, governs TEFCA, and enforces the information blocking provisions of the 21st Century Cures Act.

PDSA (Plan-Do-Study-Act) — An iterative quality improvement cycle developed by W. Edwards Deming and widely used in healthcare. The Plan phase defines the change and how to test it; Do is the small-scale pilot; Study analyzes the results against predictions; Act decides whether to adopt, adapt, or abandon the change and begins the next cycle.

Population Health — An approach to healthcare that focuses on the health outcomes of groups of individuals, including the distribution of outcomes within and across groups, and on the policies and interventions that link multiple determinants of health. In analytics, population health management uses data to identify high-risk patients, track preventive care gaps, and measure intervention effectiveness at the group level.

Prevalence — An epidemiological measure of the proportion of a population that has a particular condition at a specific point in time (point prevalence) or over a defined period (period prevalence). Prevalence reflects the existing burden of disease and is affected by both the incidence of new cases and the duration of the illness.

Primary Key — In relational database design, a column or set of columns that uniquely identifies each row in a table. Primary keys enforce entity integrity, prevent duplicate records, and serve as the basis for relational joins.

Every table in a well-designed relational schema must have a primary key; surrogate keys (system-generated integers) are commonly used when no natural unique identifier exists.

Protected Health Information (PHI) — Under HIPAA, individually identifiable health information that is transmitted or maintained by a covered entity or business associate in any form or medium, including electronic, paper, and oral. PHI includes 18 categories of identifiers defined in the HIPAA Privacy Rule, ranging from names and dates to device identifiers and full-face photographs.

Proxy Access — The authorization granted to a person (proxy) to access another individual's health information in a patient portal or health IT system, typically used for parents managing minor children's records, caregivers managing elderly patients' records, or patients designating trusted representatives. Proxy access policies must balance convenience with privacy protections.

Quality Measure — A standardized mechanism for assessing the performance of a healthcare provider, plan, or system against a defined standard of care. Quality measures are categorized as structure (resources and systems), process (whether recommended actions were performed), outcome (patient results), and patient experience. Quality measures drive value-based payment models and public reporting.

QRDA (Quality Reporting Document Architecture) — An HL7 standard for packaging clinical quality measure data for submission to CMS and other reporting programs. QRDA Category I contains patient-level data; QRDA Category III contains aggregate measure results. Both formats use XML and are required for eCQM submission under Medicare quality reporting programs.

Real-World Evidence (RWE) — Clinical evidence about the usage and potential benefits or risks of a medical product derived from real-world data (RWD) such as EHRs, claims, registries, and patient-generated data, as distinct from data collected in controlled clinical trials. The FDA and CMS increasingly recognize RWE for regulatory and coverage decisions.

Registry — A structured database used to collect and analyze standardized health data on patients with a defined condition, procedure, exposure, or demographic characteristic. Clinical registries (e.g., cancer registries, cardiac registries) support quality improvement, surveillance, research, and public health monitoring. Data are collected prospectively or through ongoing abstraction.

Risk Adjustment — A statistical methodology that accounts for differences in patient health status and demographic characteristics when comparing health outcomes, costs, or quality measures across providers, plans, or populations. Risk adjustment prevents penalizing providers who care for sicker or higher-risk patients. CMS uses HCC-based risk scores for Medicare Advantage payment.

Risk Stratification — The process of categorizing a patient population into tiers based on their likelihood of future adverse events (hospitalizations, ED visits, high costs) to prioritize care management resources. Risk stratification models may use claims, EHR, SDOH, and behavioral data and are central to population health management programs.

ROI (Release of Information) — The process by which a healthcare organization discloses a patient's protected health information to authorized requestors in accordance with HIPAA, state law, and organizational policy. ROI analysts process requests from patients, attorneys, insurers, other providers, and public health agencies, applying minimum necessary and authorization requirements.

Scrubbing — In revenue cycle management, the process of reviewing claims for errors, missing information, or payer-specific edit failures before submission. Claim scrubbing (claim editing) is performed by software that checks for correct coding, covered diagnosis-procedure combinations, invalid code pairs (CCI edits), and required field completeness to reduce denials.

SDOH (Social Determinants of Health) — The conditions in the environments where people are born, live, learn, work, play, worship, and age that affect a wide range of health and quality-of-life risks and outcomes. SDOH domains include economic stability, education, social and community context, health and health care access, and neighborhood and built environment. SDOH data are increasingly integrated into analytics for equity and population health.

Sensitivity (Statistical) — Also called recall or true positive rate, sensitivity measures a test's or model's ability to correctly identify individuals who have the condition or outcome of interest: Sensitivity = True Positives ÷ (True Positives + False Negatives). A highly sensitive test misses few true cases but may produce more false positives.

SMART on FHIR — An open, standards-based authorization framework that enables third-party applications to securely access FHIR-compliant EHR data using OAuth 2.0 and OpenID Connect. SMART (Substitutable Medical Applications, Reusable Technologies) allows apps to launch within the EHR context with scoped permissions to specific FHIR resources, supporting patient access and clinical workflow integration.

Specificity (Statistical) — Also called the true negative rate, specificity measures a test's or model's ability to correctly identify individuals who do not have the condition or outcome of interest: Specificity = True Negatives ÷ (True Negatives + False Positives). A highly specific test produces few false alarms but may miss some true cases. Sensitivity and specificity represent a fundamental trade-off in diagnostic and predictive analytics.

SQL (Structured Query Language) — The standard programming language used to manage and query relational databases. SQL supports data definition (CREATE, ALTER, DROP), data manipulation (SELECT, INSERT, UPDATE, DELETE), and data control (GRANT, REVOKE) operations. Healthcare analysts use SQL to extract, transform, and analyze data from EHR databases, claims repositories, and data warehouses.

Star Schema — A dimensional data modeling pattern used in data warehouses in which a central fact table (containing measurable events and foreign keys) is surrounded by denormalized dimension tables (describing the who, what, where, and when). The resulting diagram resembles a star. Star schemas are optimized for analytical query performance and are the most common EDW design in healthcare.

Stratification — The process of dividing a population into subgroups (strata) based on defined characteristics (age, sex, race/ethnicity, payer, geography) to compare outcomes across groups and identify disparities. Stratified reporting is a key method for health equity analytics and is required by CMS for many quality measure submissions.

TEFCA (Trusted Exchange Framework and Common Agreement) — An ONC initiative that establishes a common governance and technical framework for nationwide health information exchange. TEFCA enables any authorized participant to exchange health information with any other participant through a network of Qualified Health Information Networks (QHINs), regardless of their technology platform or location.

USCDI (United States Core Data for Interoperability) — A standardized set of health data classes and constituent data elements with broad support for interoperability in the U.S. health care system. Maintained by ONC, USCDI defines minimum data elements that certified EHRs must be capable of exchanging. Version 3 (2022) added SDOH data elements; USCDI evolves through an annual update cycle.

Value-Based Care — A healthcare delivery model in which providers are compensated based on patient health outcomes and quality of care rather than the volume of services rendered. Value-based payment models include ACOs, bundled payments, quality bonus programs, and pay-for-performance arrangements. Analytics are central to tracking performance and identifying improvement opportunities.

Variance — In statistics, a measure of the spread or dispersion of data values around the mean, calculated as the average of squared deviations from the mean. In healthcare operations, "variance" also refers to the difference between expected (budgeted or benchmarked) and actual performance on a metric such as cost, LOS, or utilization. Variance analysis identifies root causes of performance gaps.

Vital Statistics — Official data on births, deaths, fetal deaths, marriages, and divorces collected by state and local civil registration systems and compiled nationally by the National Center for Health Statistics (NCHS). Vital statistics data are used for population health surveillance, epidemiological research, cause-of-death coding, and public health policy. Death certificates are a primary source of mortality data in the U.S.

Workflow Analysis — A systematic examination of the sequence of tasks, decision points, roles, and information flows involved in a work process to identify inefficiencies, bottlenecks, redundancies, and opportunities for improvement. In health IT and HIM, workflow analysis is conducted before EHR implementation, data governance redesign, or quality improvement initiatives to ensure that technology supports rather than disrupts care delivery.

.43 Appendix A: Quick Reference — Statistical Formulas and Healthcare Metrics

This appendix consolidates the core statistical formulas and healthcare-specific metrics that appear throughout the CHDA examination. Each entry includes the formula, a definition of all variables, and a concise note on its applied use in health data analytics practice.

1. Mean (Arithmetic Mean)

Formula: $\bar{x} = (\Sigma x_i) / n$

Variables: $\bar{x}$ = mean; x_i = each individual value in the dataset; n = total number of observations; Σ = summation operator.

Clinical/Analytics Use: Calculating the average length of stay across a patient population to benchmark against regional or national norms.

2. Median

Formula: For an ordered dataset of n values, Median = value at position $(n + 1) / 2$ when n is odd; average of values at positions $n/2$ and $(n/2 + 1)$ when n is even.

Variables: n = total number of observations; ordered values arranged from smallest to largest.

Clinical/Analytics Use: Reporting the middle value of hospital charges, which is preferred over the mean when cost distributions are heavily right-skewed by outlier cases.

3. Mode

Formula: Mode = the value(s) that appear with the highest frequency in a dataset.

Variables: No algebraic formula; determined by frequency count of each distinct value.

Clinical/Analytics Use: Identifying the most frequently assigned ICD-10-CM diagnosis code in an outpatient clinic to prioritize documentation training.

4. Standard Deviation

Formula (population): $\sigma = \sqrt{[\, \Sigma(x_i - \mu)^2 / N \,]}$ Formula (sample): $s = \sqrt{[\, \Sigma(x_i - \bar{x})^2 / (n - 1) \,]}$

Variables: σ = population standard deviation; s = sample standard deviation; x_i = each observation; μ = population mean; $\bar{x}$ = sample mean; N = population size; n = sample size.

Clinical/Analytics Use: Measuring variability in patient wait times to identify whether a department consistently performs near its average or has wide, unpredictable fluctuations.

5. Variance

Formula (population): $\sigma^2 = \Sigma(x_i - \mu)^2 / N$ Formula (sample): $s^2 = \Sigma(x_i - \bar{x})^2 / (n - 1)$

Variables: σ^2 = population variance; s^2 = sample variance; all other variables as defined for standard deviation.

Clinical/Analytics Use: Comparing variance in procedure costs across multiple service lines to identify which line shows the greatest financial unpredictability.

6. Coefficient of Variation (CV)

Formula: $CV = (s / \bar{x}) \times 100$

Variables: CV = coefficient of variation expressed as a percentage; s = sample standard deviation; $\bar{x}$ = sample mean.

Clinical/Analytics Use: Comparing variability in resource utilization between departments with different average costs, enabling fair cross-departmental comparison on a standardized scale.

7. Prevalence Rate

Formula: Prevalence Rate = (Number of existing cases of condition at a point in time / Total population at risk at that time) × 10□

Variables: 10□ = multiplier (commonly 1,000 or 100,000) chosen to yield a meaningful rate; numerator = existing cases; denominator = population at risk.

Clinical/Analytics Use: Estimating the burden of diabetes in a health system's attributed population to plan disease management program capacity.

8. Incidence Rate

Formula: Incidence Rate = (Number of new cases during a specified period / Population at risk during that period) × 10□

Variables: Numerator = newly diagnosed cases; denominator = person-time at risk or midpoint population; 10□ = scaling multiplier.

Clinical/Analytics Use: Tracking the rate of new hospital-acquired infections per 1,000 patient-days to measure the effectiveness of an infection prevention intervention.

9. Sensitivity (True Positive Rate)

Formula: Sensitivity = TP / (TP + FN)

Variables: TP = true positives (disease present, test positive); FN = false negatives (disease present, test negative); TP + FN = all individuals who actually have the condition.

Clinical/Analytics Use: Evaluating a screening algorithm's ability to correctly identify all patients with a high-risk condition so that no true cases are missed.

10. Specificity (True Negative Rate)

Formula: Specificity = TN / (TN + FP)

Variables: TN = true negatives (disease absent, test negative); FP = false positives (disease absent, test positive); TN + FP = all individuals who actually do not have the condition.

Clinical/Analytics Use: Assessing a predictive model's ability to correctly exclude patients who do not have a condition, minimizing unnecessary follow-up interventions.

11. Positive Predictive Value (PPV)

Formula: PPV = TP / (TP + FP)

Variables: TP = true positives; FP = false positives; TP + FP = all positive test results.

Clinical/Analytics Use: Determining what proportion of patients flagged as high-risk by a readmission prediction tool actually are readmitted, informing the practical utility of the tool.

12. Negative Predictive Value (NPV)

Formula: NPV = TN / (TN + FN)

Variables: TN = true negatives; FN = false negatives; TN + FN = all negative test results.

Clinical/Analytics Use: Assessing confidence that a patient who screens negative for a condition is truly disease-free, which is critical for determining the safety of a rule-out strategy.

13. Relative Risk (Risk Ratio)

Formula: RR = [a / (a + b)] / [c / (c + d)]

Variables: a = exposed with disease; b = exposed without disease; c = unexposed with disease; d = unexposed without disease; a/(a+b) = incidence in exposed group; c/(c+d) = incidence in unexposed group.

Clinical/Analytics Use: Comparing the likelihood of a surgical complication between patients who received a prophylactic antibiotic versus those who did not.

14. Odds Ratio (OR)

Formula: OR = (a × d) / (b × c)

Variables: Using the standard 2×2 contingency table: a = exposed cases; b = exposed non-cases; c = unexposed cases; d = unexposed non-cases.

Clinical/Analytics Use: Quantifying the association between a risk factor (such as smoking) and a health outcome in a case-control study drawn from retrospective health records.

15. Number Needed to Treat (NNT)

Formula: NNT = 1 / ARR, where ARR = Control Event Rate − Experimental Event Rate

Variables: ARR = absolute risk reduction; Control Event Rate = proportion of adverse events in the control group; Experimental Event Rate = proportion of adverse events in the treatment group.

Clinical/Analytics Use: Communicating how many patients must receive a new care protocol before one additional adverse event is prevented, translating statistical efficacy into clinical significance.

16. Average Daily Census (ADC)

Formula: ADC = Total Inpatient Service Days for a Period / Number of Days in the Period

Variables: Total Inpatient Service Days = sum of patients present at census time each day; Number of Days = length of reporting period (e.g., 30 for a month).

Clinical/Analytics Use: Benchmarking daily patient volume to assess staffing adequacy and compare occupancy across departments or facilities.

17. Average Length of Stay (ALOS)

Formula: ALOS = Total Inpatient Service Days / Total Discharges

Variables: Total Inpatient Service Days = sum of all patient-days within the period; Total Discharges = number of patients discharged (including deaths) in the same period.

Clinical/Analytics Use: Comparing a facility's ALOS against payer benchmarks or DRG expected values to identify potential opportunities for care coordination improvements.

18. Occupancy Rate

Formula: Occupancy Rate = (ADC / Bed Count) × 100

Variables: ADC = average daily census; Bed Count = number of licensed beds (or staffed beds, depending on the reporting standard applied).

Clinical/Analytics Use: Evaluating how efficiently a hospital is utilizing its inpatient capacity, where rates below 60% may indicate underutilization and above 85% may signal access constraints.

19. Bed Turnover Rate

Formula: Bed Turnover Rate = Total Discharges / Average Bed Count

Variables: Total Discharges = number of patients discharged in the period; Average Bed Count = average number of available beds during the same period.

Clinical/Analytics Use: Measuring how many times per period an average bed is occupied by a discharged patient, which reflects the throughput efficiency of the unit.

20. Crude Mortality Rate

Formula: Crude Mortality Rate = (Total Deaths in a Population During a Period / Total Midperiod Population) × 10□

Variables: Numerator = all deaths from any cause; Denominator = estimated population at the midpoint of the period; 10□ = typically 1,000 or 100,000.

Clinical/Analytics Use: Comparing overall death rates across counties or health service areas as an initial population health surveillance measure before age-adjustment is applied.

21. Case Fatality Rate (CFR)

Formula: CFR = (Deaths Due to a Specific Disease / Confirmed Cases of That Disease) × 100

Variables: Deaths = fatalities directly attributed to the disease within a defined period; Confirmed Cases = total diagnosed cases of the disease in the same period.

Clinical/Analytics Use: Monitoring the lethality of a disease outbreak or tracking mortality outcomes for a specific diagnosis within a hospital's case mix.

22. Standardized Mortality Ratio (SMR)

Formula: SMR = (Observed Deaths / Expected Deaths) × 100

Variables: Observed Deaths = actual number of deaths in the study population; Expected Deaths = number of deaths that would be expected if the study population had the same age-specific (and optionally sex-specific) death rates as the reference population.

Clinical/Analytics Use: Comparing a hospital's or region's mortality experience against a national reference standard while controlling for differences in the age distribution of the populations.

23. Readmission Rate

Formula: Readmission Rate = (Number of Readmissions Within a Defined Window / Total Discharges in the Denominator Population) × 100

Variables: Readmission Window = typically 30, 60, or 90 days post-discharge; Denominator Population = index discharges meeting eligibility criteria (often excludes planned readmissions and certain DRGs per CMS methodology).

Clinical/Analytics Use: Tracking 30-day all-cause readmission rates as a quality and value metric under CMS Hospital Readmissions Reduction Program (HRRP) reporting requirements.

24. Complication Rate

Formula: Complication Rate = (Number of Cases with One or More Complications / Total Cases in the Study Group) × 100

Variables: Complications = adverse events occurring after the primary procedure or diagnosis, often defined by POA (present on admission) indicator or PSI (patient safety indicator) methodology; Total Cases = all eligible discharges in the period and group.

Clinical/Analytics Use: Benchmarking surgical complication rates by surgeon, service line, or facility to target quality improvement efforts and risk-adjust performance comparisons.

25. Case Mix Index (CMI)

Formula: CMI = Σ(DRG Relative Weight × Number of Cases in That DRG) / Total Cases Equivalently: CMI = Sum of All DRG Relative Weights for Discharged Cases / Total Discharges

Variables: DRG Relative Weight = CMS-assigned resource intensity weight for each MS-DRG; Number of Cases = discharges falling into each DRG; Total Cases = all discharges included in the calculation period.

Clinical/Analytics Use: Measuring the complexity and resource intensity of a hospital's inpatient population, which directly determines Medicare reimbursement and is used to adjust quality comparisons across facilities with different patient acuity profiles.

CHDA Exam Domain Crosswalk

The AHIMA CHDA examination is organized into seven domains reflecting the competencies required of a practicing health data analyst. The table below maps each domain to its examination weight, primary topics, relevant chapters in this study guide, and high-yield terminology that frequently appears on the exam.

Domain	Domain Name	Exam Weight	Key Topics Tested	Recommended Chapters	High-Yield Exam Terms
1	Data Management and Governance	20%	Data governance frameworks; data stewardship roles and responsibilities; data quality dimensions (accuracy, completeness, consistency, timeliness, validity, uniqueness); metadata management; master patient index (MPI); data dictionaries; data lifecycle management; regulatory compliance (HIPAA, 21st Century Cures Act); data retention policies; enterprise data governance structures	Chapters 1–2	Data steward; data governance council; data provenance; metadata; MPI; data quality dimensions; data dictionary; chain of custody; de-identification; limited data set

Domain	Domain Name	Exam Weight	Key Topics Tested	Recommended Chapters	High-Yield Exam Terms
2	Data Analytics and Statistical Methods	22%	Descriptive, inferential, and predictive analytics; parametric vs. non-parametric tests; hypothesis testing (null/alternative hypothesis, p-value, confidence intervals); regression analysis (linear, logistic, multiple); correlation coefficients; chi-square tests; t-tests and ANOVA; survival analysis; time-series analysis; risk adjustment methodologies; sampling methods; power and sample size; Type I and Type II error	Chapters 3–4	p-value; confidence interval; statistical significance; regression coefficient; odds ratio; relative risk; sensitivity; specificity; Type I error (alpha); Type II error (beta); power; Pearson r; Spearman rho
3	Data Visualization and Reporting	14%	Selection of appropriate chart types for data types and audiences; dashboard design principles; run charts and control charts (SPC); Pareto charts; heat maps; scatter plots; geographic information systems (GIS); data storytelling; report design for executive vs. operational audiences; visualization tools and platforms; use of color, accessibility, and clarity standards	Chapters 5–6	Control chart; run chart; special cause variation; common cause variation; upper control limit (UCL); lower control limit (LCL); dashboard; KPI; Pareto principle; SPC; data story

Domain	Domain Name	Exam Weight	Key Topics Tested	Recommended Chapters	High-Yield Exam Terms
4	Health Data and Information Management	16%	Healthcare data sources (EHR, claims, registries, surveys, PROs); UB-04 and CMS-1500 claim forms; ICD-10-CM/PCS and CPT coding and data use; DRG assignment and grouper logic; present on admission (POA) indicators; revenue cycle data elements; HIM functions supporting analytics; secondary data sources; national databases (NHDS, NIS, HCUP, BRFSS, Vital Statistics); health information exchange (HIE)	Chapters 7–8	MS-DRG; APR-DRG; principal diagnosis; POA indicator; CC/MCC; HCC; UB-04; revenue code; HCUP; NHIS; BRFSS; HIE; ADT; HL7; FHIR

Domain	Domain Name	Exam Weight	Key Topics Tested	Recommended Chapters	High-Yield Exam Terms
5	Research Methods and Evidence-Based Practice	12%	Research design types (RCT, cohort, case-control, cross-sectional, ecological); internal and external validity; confounding variables and effect modification; bias types (selection, information, recall, Hawthorne effect); systematic review and meta-analysis methods; IRB and research ethics; CONSORT and STROBE reporting standards; translating research into practice; levels of evidence hierarchy; pragmatic vs. explanatory trials	Chapters 9–10	Internal validity; external validity; confounding; selection bias; information bias; IRB; CONSORT; STROBE; intent-to-treat; per-protocol; levels of evidence; systematic review; meta-analysis

Domain	Domain Name	Exam Weight	Key Topics Tested	Recommended Chapters	High-Yield Exam Terms
6	Quality and Performance Improvement	10%	CMS quality programs (HRRP, VBP, HAC Reduction Program, MIPS/APMs); Joint Commission performance measurement standards; NCQA HEDIS measures; core measures; patient safety indicators (PSIs) and hospital-acquired conditions (HACs); PDSA cycle; Lean and Six Sigma in healthcare; root cause analysis; failure mode and effects analysis (FMEA); benchmarking methodologies; outcome vs. process vs. structural measures	Chapters 10–11	HRRP; VBP; HAC; PSI; HEDIS; PDSA; Lean; Six Sigma; DMAIC; FMEA; root cause analysis; sentinel event; core measure; never event; Donabedian model

Domain	Domain Name	Exam Weight	Key Topics Tested	Recommended Chapters	High-Yield Exam Terms
7	Health Information Technology and Systems	6%	EHR systems and certification standards (ONC, 2015 Edition); interoperability standards (HL7 v2, HL7 FHIR, CDA, C-CDA); clinical decision support systems; natural language processing (NLP) in HIM; health information exchanges; cloud computing in healthcare; cybersecurity fundamentals (HIPAA Security Rule, risk analysis); telehealth data considerations; emerging technologies (AI, machine learning in clinical analytics); APIs and data integration	Chapters 11–12	FHIR; HL7; C-CDA; ONC; interoperability; NLP; CDS; API; risk analysis; HIPAA Security Rule; encryption; cloud security; telehealth

Notes on Using This Crosswalk:

1. Domain weights reflect the approximate proportion of scored questions on the 180-item examination. Domains 1 and 2 together account for 42% of the exam, making statistical fluency and data governance the highest-priority preparation areas.
2. High-yield exam terms are terms that have appeared consistently across multiple released AHIMA practice examinations and candidate reports. Ensure you can define each term, distinguish it from closely related terms, and apply it in a brief scenario.
3. Chapter references in this guide are approximate; many topics span multiple chapters. When a topic appears in both the crosswalk and the Chapter Review Questions, prioritize that intersection for final review.
4. AHIMA periodically revises domain weights following job task analyses. Candidates should verify current domain weights against the official CHDA Candidate Guide available at ahima.org before scheduling their examination.

CHDA Study Schedules

Two structured study schedules are provided below. Choose the schedule that best matches your background and available preparation time. Both schedules assume access to this study guide, a practice question bank with at least 300 CHDA-aligned questions, and a notes system (digital or paper) for active recall practice.

.44 4-Week Intensive Schedule

Designed for candidates who hold an active RHIA or RHIT credential, have prior experience working with health data analytics tools, and are comfortable with foundational statistics. Target study time: 2–3 hours per day on weekdays; 4–5 hours per day on weekends.

.44.1 Week 1: Data Foundations and Statistical Core

Monday — Day 1 Read: Chapter 1 (Data Management and Governance Overview) in full. Practice Questions: Complete 20 questions from Domain 1. Activity: Create a one-page summary of the six data quality dimensions with a healthcare example for each.

Tuesday — Day 2 Read: Chapter 2 (Data Governance Frameworks and Regulatory Compliance). Practice Questions: Complete 20 questions from Domain 1. Activity: Draw a diagram of a hospital enterprise data governance structure, including the data governance council, data stewards, and subject matter domains.

Wednesday — Day 3 Read: Chapter 3, Part 1 (Descriptive Statistics and Distributions). Practice Questions: Complete 25 questions from Domain 2, focusing on descriptive statistics. Activity: Work through all 25 formulas in Appendix A by hand, identifying which you can reproduce from memory and which require additional review.

Thursday — Day 4 Read: Chapter 3, Part 2 (Inferential Statistics: Hypothesis Testing and Confidence Intervals). Practice Questions: Complete 25 questions from Domain 2, focusing on hypothesis testing concepts. Activity: Write out the four steps of hypothesis testing (state hypotheses, select significance level, calculate test statistic, draw conclusion) and practice applying them to two sample healthcare scenarios.

Friday — Day 5 Read: Chapter 4 (Regression Analysis and Predictive Methods). Practice Questions: Complete 20 questions from Domain 2, focusing on regression and correlation. Activity: Review Type I and Type II error definitions; create a 2×2 matrix contrasting them with their consequences in clinical analytics contexts.

Saturday — Day 6 Review: Re-read flagged sections from Days 1–5. Review all incorrect practice question answers, tracing each error to a specific knowledge gap. Practice Questions: Complete a timed 40-question mixed block from Domains 1 and 2. Target completion in 50 minutes. Activity: Update your formula summary sheet with any gaps identified during the week.

Sunday — Day 7 Rest or light review only. Optional: Watch one educational video or listen to a podcast on a statistical topic that felt unclear during the week. No new material.

.44.2 Week 2: Healthcare Data, Visualization, and Reporting

Monday — Day 8 Read: Chapter 7 (Healthcare Data Sources and the Revenue Cycle). Practice Questions: Complete 20 questions from Domain 4. Activity: Sketch the flow of a patient encounter from registration through claims submission, labeling each data element captured at each stage.

Tuesday — Day 9 Read: Chapter 8 (Coding Systems, DRG Logic, and Secondary Data). Practice Questions: Complete 20 questions from Domain 4. Activity: Create a comparison table of MS-DRG vs. APR-DRG methodologies, including their primary use cases and the role of CC/MCC designations.

Wednesday — Day 10 Read: Chapter 5 (Data Visualization Principles and Chart Selection). Practice Questions: Complete 20 questions from Domain 3. Activity: For each of the following data types—trend over time, distribution, comparison of categories, correlation between two variables, and geographic distribution—identify the single most appropriate visualization type and explain why.

Thursday — Day 11 Read: Chapter 6 (Statistical Process Control and Dashboard Design). Practice Questions: Complete 20 questions from Domain 3. Activity: Interpret a provided run chart: identify the centerline, mark any runs of eight or more consecutive points above or below the centerline, and classify whether special cause variation is present.

Friday — Day 12 Read: Chapter 9 (Research Design and Evidence-Based Practice). Practice Questions: Complete 25 questions from Domain 5. Activity: Create a hierarchy-of-evidence pyramid (systematic review/meta-analysis at top through expert opinion at bottom) and assign one healthcare analytics example to each level.

Saturday — Day 13 Review: Timed 50-question mixed block from Domains 3, 4, and 5. Target 60 minutes. Practice Questions: Review all incorrect answers. Categorize errors as conceptual gaps, terminology confusion, or calculation errors. Address each category differently in subsequent days. Activity: Complete the Domain Crosswalk table in Appendix B: for each high-yield term you marked as uncertain, write a one-sentence definition without looking at the text.

Sunday — Day 14 Rest or light review. Optional: Visit the AHIMA website to review any recently posted CHDA exam candidate information or errata.

.44.3 Week 3: Quality Improvement, Research Methods, and HIT

Monday — Day 15 Read: Chapter 10 (Quality and Performance Improvement Programs). Practice Questions: Complete 25 questions from Domain 6. Activity: Map the CMS quality programs covered on the exam (HRRP, VBP, HAC Reduction, MIPS/APMs) to their legislative origins, metrics, and financial consequences.

Tuesday — Day 16 Read: Chapter 11, Part 1 (PDSA, Lean, Six Sigma, and Root Cause Analysis). Practice Questions: Complete 20 questions from Domain 6. Activity: Draft a sample PDSA cycle for a hypothetical quality problem (e.g., reducing catheter-associated urinary tract infections) by filling in each of the four phases with specific, concrete steps.

Wednesday — Day 17 Read: Chapter 11, Part 2 (Health Information Technology and Interoperability). Practice Questions: Complete 20 questions from Domain 7. Activity: Build a terminology comparison table: HL7 v2 vs. FHIR — include year of introduction, primary use case, message format, and current adoption context.

Thursday — Day 18 Read: Chapter 12 (Cybersecurity, Privacy, and Emerging Technologies in Health Analytics). Practice Questions: Complete 20 questions from Domain 7. Activity: List the five required components of a HIPAA Security Rule risk analysis and write one sentence on how each component would be documented in a real health analytics environment.

Friday — Day 19 Mixed Review: Re-read the summary sections at the end of Chapters 9, 10, 11, and 12. Practice Questions: Complete a timed 60-question mixed block drawn proportionally from all seven domains. Score and record the result. Activity: Identify your two lowest-scoring domains from this block. Schedule targeted review of those domains on Saturday.

Saturday — Day 20 Targeted Review: Focus exclusively on the two weakest domains identified on Friday. Re-read relevant chapters, redo missed questions, and create flashcards for any terms that remain uncertain. Practice Questions: Complete 30 additional questions in the two targeted domains. Activity: Revisit the formulas in Appendix A that you could not reproduce from memory in Week 1 and attempt them again without reference.

Sunday — Day 21 Rest. No new material. Prepare your exam-day materials: confirm exam location (or remote testing setup), gather required identification, and review any AHIMA candidate handbook requirements.

.44.4 Week 4: Integration and Final Preparation

Monday — Day 22 Full Practice Exam: Complete a full-length 180-question timed practice exam (target: 3 hours 45 minutes). Use a practice question bank configured to mirror CHDA domain proportions. Activity: After scoring, categorize all incorrect answers by domain. This analysis drives the remainder of Week 4.

Tuesday — Day 23 Targeted Weak-Domain Remediation: Spend the day on your two or three lowest-scoring domains from Monday's practice exam. Re-read the relevant chapters and complete 30–40 domain-specific questions. Activity: For each incorrect answer on Monday's exam, write a one-line explanation of the correct reasoning in your own words.

Wednesday — Day 24 Mixed Review: Complete 60 questions across all domains at timed pace. Activity: Review all statistical formulas in Appendix A; time yourself reproducing each formula from scratch in under 30 seconds. Flag any that still require rehearsal. Review: Scan the Domain Crosswalk in Appendix B and verbally define each high-yield term without looking at the definition.

Thursday — Day 25 Light Review: Read only the chapter summary boxes and key term lists at the end of each chapter. Practice Questions: Complete 40 questions at a relaxed pace, focusing on understanding rationale rather than speed. Activity: Review your personal notes, formula sheet, and any flashcards you have created. Do not attempt to learn new material at this stage.

Friday — Day 26 Rest Day: No practice questions. No new material. Engage in a relaxing, non-academic activity. Logistics Confirmation: Confirm your exam appointment, testing center address or remote proctoring setup, required identification documents, and any materials restrictions.

Saturday — Day 27 Light Review (Morning Only): Spend no more than 90 minutes reviewing the Appendix A formula sheet and the high-yield terms in Appendix B. Stop by noon. Afternoon/Evening: Rest completely. Eat a nutritious meal, avoid alcohol, and prioritize sleep. Aim for 7–8 hours before exam day.

Sunday — Day 28 — Exam Day Morning: Eat a substantial breakfast. Arrive at the testing center 30 minutes early, or log into the remote proctoring platform 15 minutes before your appointment window opens. During the Exam: Flag uncertain questions and return to them after completing the full exam. Pace yourself at approximately 1.25 minutes per question. Do not spend more than 2 minutes on any single question on the first pass. After the Exam: Record your impressions about which domains felt strongest and weakest; these notes may be useful if you need to retake the examination.

.45 8-Week Comprehensive Schedule

Designed for candidates who are newer to health data analytics, may not hold an RHIA or RHIT, or who benefit from extended review time and spaced repetition. Target study time: 1.5–2 hours per day on weekdays; 3–4 hours per day on weekends.

.45.1 Week 1: Prerequisite and Foundation Review

This week is reserved for closing any knowledge gaps in prerequisite areas before beginning domain-specific content. If you are confident in all areas below, use this week to begin Week 2 content and add one additional week to any later phase.

Monday — Day 1 Prerequisite Review: Basic math review — fractions, percentages, ratios, and proportions. Verify you can convert between these forms rapidly and accurately without a calculator. Activity: Complete 10 basic math problems representative of healthcare rate calculations (e.g., calculating a percentage of a total, converting a rate per 1,000 to a decimal). Correct all errors before moving on.

Tuesday — Day 2 Prerequisite Review: Introduction to healthcare terminology — review primary, secondary, and tertiary care settings; inpatient vs. outpatient distinctions; acute, post-acute, and ambulatory care definitions. Activity: Create a one-page glossary of 30 healthcare setting and care delivery terms you expect to encounter on the exam.

Wednesday — Day 3 Prerequisite Review: Introduction to the healthcare revenue cycle — overview of the patient financial journey from registration through payer adjudication, including the roles of charge capture, coding, billing, and claims processing. Activity: Sketch the revenue cycle workflow and label the primary data touchpoints where health data analysts interact with financial and clinical data.

Thursday — Day 4 Prerequisite Review: Introduction to health information management — the role of HIM professionals; the transition from paper to electronic health records; core HIM functions (coding, release of information, record completion, compliance). Activity: Read the AHIMA CHDA competency framework summary (available at ahima.org) and align each competency to one of the seven exam domains.

Friday — Day 5 Prerequisite Review: Introduction to regulatory environment — HIPAA (Privacy Rule, Security Rule, Breach Notification Rule), the 21st Century Cures Act, and CMS quality reporting programs at a high level. Activity: Write a one-paragraph summary of each of the three HIPAA rules in plain language, as if explaining to a colleague who is not in healthcare.

Saturday — Day 6 Review: Revisit any prerequisite area from Days 1–5 that felt uncertain. Begin reading Chapter 1 of this guide (Data Management and Governance). Activity: Complete the self-assessment at the end of Chapter 1 and record your score for baseline tracking.

Sunday — Day 7 Rest. Optional light reading only.

.45.2 Week 2: Data Management and Governance (Domain 1)

Monday — Day 8 Read: Chapter 1 in full at a careful pace, pausing to take notes on each major concept. Practice Questions: Complete 15 questions from Domain 1. Activity: Create a flashcard set for the six data quality dimensions. On each card: term on front, definition plus one healthcare example on back.

Tuesday — Day 9 Read: Chapter 2 (Data Governance Frameworks and Regulatory Compliance). Practice Questions: Complete 15 questions from Domain 1. Activity: Compare and contrast the roles of a data steward and a data governance council in a hospital setting, using a two-column format.

Wednesday — Day 10 Review: Re-read flagged sections from Chapters 1 and 2. Practice Questions: Complete a 30-question mixed Domain 1 block. Activity: Review all incorrect answers and trace each error to a chapter section. Re-read those sections before Thursday.

Thursday — Day 11 Spaced Repetition: Without opening the book, write down everything you remember about data governance structures, data quality dimensions, and HIPAA compliance requirements. Then check your notes against the text and identify gaps. Practice Questions: Complete 20 additional Domain 1 questions. Activity: Update your flashcard set with any terms that appeared in practice questions but were not in your original set.

Friday — Day 12 Light review of Domain 1 material. Begin previewing Chapter 3 headings and summary boxes. Practice Questions: Complete 15 Domain 1 questions for reinforcement. Activity: Rest. Domain 1 review is complete for the primary cycle; it will return in spaced repetition cycles during Weeks 5 and 7.

Saturday — Day 13 Read: Chapter 3, Part 1 (Descriptive Statistics). Activity: Work through the first 10 formulas in Appendix A by hand. Write out each formula, define the variables, and calculate a sample result using invented but realistic numbers. Practice Questions: 20 Domain 2 questions on descriptive statistics.

Sunday — Day 14 Rest or light review of statistics flash cards.

.45.3 Week 3: Statistics and Analytical Methods (Domain 2, Part 1)

Monday — Day 15 Read: Chapter 3, Part 2 (Inferential Statistics and Hypothesis Testing). Practice Questions: Complete 20 Domain 2 questions. Activity: Diagram the decision tree for choosing between a t-test, chi-square test, and ANOVA based on the number of groups and the level of measurement of the outcome variable.

Tuesday — Day 16 Read: Chapter 4, Part 1 (Correlation and Linear Regression). Practice Questions: Complete 20 Domain 2 questions. Activity: Work through Appendix A formulas 13–15 (relative risk, odds ratio, NNT). Create a side-by-side comparison of when each is used and what study designs they are associated with.

Wednesday — Day 17 Read: Chapter 4, Part 2 (Logistic Regression and Predictive Modeling Concepts). Practice Questions: Complete 20 Domain 2 questions. Activity: Summarize the assumptions of linear regression and the circumstances under which logistic regression is the more appropriate choice.

Thursday — Day 18 Read: Chapter 4, Part 3 (Risk Adjustment and Standardization Methods). Practice Questions: Complete 20 Domain 2 questions. Activity: Work through the SMR formula (Appendix A, item 22) and the CMI formula (item 25) by hand, using sample data.

Friday — Day 19 Spaced Repetition: Return to Domain 1 material without looking at notes. Reconstruct from memory the primary elements of a data governance framework. Check against your Week 2 notes. Record any persistent gaps. Practice Questions: Complete a 40-question mixed block from Domains 1 and 2. Activity: Score and record results. Calculate your accuracy percentage for each domain separately.

Saturday — Day 20 Targeted Review: Address any Domain 2 weaknesses identified in Friday's mixed block. Practice Questions: 25 additional Domain 2 questions. Activity: Begin building a cumulative formula reference sheet from Appendix A, written entirely from memory. Compare against Appendix A and fill in gaps.

Sunday — Day 21 Rest.

.45.4 Week 4: Healthcare Data and Health Information Management (Domain 4)

Monday — Day 22 Read: Chapter 7 in full (Healthcare Data Sources and the Revenue Cycle). Practice Questions: Complete 20 Domain 4 questions. Activity: Create a table listing 10 national health data sources (e.g., HCUP, BRFSS, NHDS, Vital Statistics, SEER) with columns for sponsoring organization, data type, unit of analysis, and primary analytic use.

Tuesday — Day 23 Read: Chapter 8, Part 1 (ICD-10-CM/PCS, CPT, and DRG Logic). Practice Questions: Complete 20 Domain 4 questions. Activity: Walk through the MS-DRG assignment logic: principal diagnosis □ MDC □ surgical/medical partition □ CC/MCC level □ specific DRG. Apply this logic to three example cases.

Wednesday — Day 24 Read: Chapter 8, Part 2 (Secondary Data Sources, HIE, and HIM Functions in Analytics). Practice Questions: Complete 20 Domain 4 questions. Activity: Compare primary and secondary data sources in a two-column table, with entries for definition, examples, advantages, and limitations in an analytics context.

Thursday — Day 25 Spaced Repetition: Return to Domains 1 and 2 briefly. Spend 30 minutes on formula recall and 30 minutes on data governance terminology flashcards. Practice Questions: Complete a 30-question mixed block from Domains 1, 2, and 4. Activity: Score and review. Identify any Domain 4 terminology that continues to produce errors and flag for Saturday review.

Friday — Day 26 Begin Visualization Content: Read Chapter 5, Part 1 (Chart Selection and Design Principles). Practice Questions: Complete 15 Domain 3 questions. Activity: For each of six chart types (bar, line, scatter, histogram, Pareto, heat map), write one sentence on the data type for which it is most appropriate.

Saturday — Day 27 Read: Chapter 5, Part 2 and Chapter 6 (SPC, Run Charts, Dashboard Design). Practice Questions: Complete 20 Domain 3 questions. Activity: Interpret a sample control chart: identify the centerline, UCL, and LCL; determine whether the process is stable; identify any rule violations indicating special cause.

Sunday — Day 28 Rest.

.45.5 Week 5: Visualization, Reporting, and Spaced Repetition Cycle 1

Monday — Day 29 Spaced Repetition Cycle 1: Domains 1, 2, and 4. Spend 30 minutes each (90 minutes total) reviewing all flagged flashcards and reworking missed practice questions from these domains without looking at answers first. Practice Questions: 30-question mixed block, Domains 1, 2, 4. Target 80% accuracy. Record result.

Tuesday — Day 30 Read: Chapter 9, Part 1 (Research Design Types and Validity). Practice Questions: Complete 20 Domain 5 questions. Activity: Create a comparison table of observational study designs (cohort, case-control, cross-sectional) with columns for temporal direction, exposure/outcome measurement sequence, typical research question, and primary threats to validity.

Wednesday — Day 31 Read: Chapter 9, Part 2 (Bias, Confounding, and Research Ethics). Practice Questions: Complete 20 Domain 5 questions. Activity: Identify one specific example of each of the following biases in a realistic healthcare data analytics scenario: selection bias, information bias, Hawthorne effect, and recall bias.

Thursday — Day 32 Read: Chapter 10, Part 1 (Evidence Hierarchy and Systematic Review Methods). Practice Questions: Complete 20 Domain 5 questions. Activity: Construct the evidence hierarchy pyramid from memory. Add one example study type to each level.

Friday — Day 33 Mixed Practice: 50-question mixed block across all domains covered to date (1, 2, 3, 4, 5). Activity: Score and record. Calculate per-domain accuracy. Flag the two domains with lowest accuracy for intensive review in Week 6.

Saturday — Day 34 Targeted Review: Address the two lowest-accuracy domains from Friday. Re-read relevant sections, rework missed questions, and update flashcard sets. Practice Questions: 30 additional questions in the two weakest domains.

Sunday — Day 35 Rest.

.45.6 Week 6: Quality Improvement, HIT, and Weak-Domain Remediation

Monday — Day 36 Read: Chapter 10, Part 2 (Quality Programs: HRRP, VBP, HAC Reduction, MIPS). Practice Questions: Complete 25 Domain 6 questions. Activity: Construct a comparison table of the four major CMS quality programs — include the program name, authorizing legislation, types of measures used, and financial mechanism (bonus or penalty).

Tuesday — Day 37 Read: Chapter 11, Part 1 (PDSA, Lean, Six Sigma, and Root Cause Analysis). Practice Questions: Complete 20 Domain 6 questions. Activity: Draft a mock root cause analysis for a hypothetical sentinel event (e.g., wrong-site surgery) using a fishbone/Ishikawa diagram format.

Wednesday — Day 38 Read: Chapter 11, Part 2 and Chapter 12 (Health IT, Interoperability, Cybersecurity). Practice Questions: Complete 20 Domain 7 questions. Activity: Summarize the differences between HL7 v2, HL7 FHIR, and CDA/C-CDA in three rows of a comparison table (format, primary use, adoption era).

Thursday — Day 39 Spaced Repetition Cycle 2: All seven domains. Spend 15 minutes per domain reviewing flashcards (105 minutes total). Flag any terms that still feel uncertain. Practice Questions: 40-question timed mixed block across all seven domains. Activity: Score and analyze. Compare per-domain accuracy to Week 5 results to measure improvement.

Friday — Day 40 Targeted Remediation: Focus on any domain where accuracy has not yet reached 70%. Re-read chapter sections and complete additional targeted practice questions. Activity: Review and drill all flagged statistical formulas using Appendix A. Target sub-30-second recall for each.

Saturday — Day 41 Full-Length Practice Exam 1: Complete a 180-question timed practice exam in exam conditions (no interruptions, no reference materials). Activity: Score and record result. Categorize all incorrect answers by domain and error type (conceptual gap, terminology, calculation, scenario misread).

Sunday — Day 42 Rest. Review practice exam results briefly to plan Week 7 priorities. No active studying.

.45.7 Week 7: Integration and Gap Closure

Monday — Day 43 Targeted Remediation: Based on Practice Exam 1 results, address your three lowest-performing domains. Re-read relevant chapter sections and complete 25–30 questions per weak domain.

Tuesday — Day 44 Targeted Remediation (continued): Address the remaining weak domains. Return to Appendix A for any formulas that appeared in Practice Exam 1 items you missed.

Wednesday — Day 45 Spaced Repetition Cycle 3: Full flashcard review across all domains. Retire any card you have answered correctly four times in a row. Focus remaining study time on unretired cards. Practice Questions: 60-question mixed block. Target 75% or higher accuracy.

Thursday — Day 46 Mixed Review: Re-read the chapter summary boxes and key term sections of every chapter in the guide. Activity: Verbally explain the Domain Crosswalk in Appendix B aloud as if teaching the material to someone else. Teaching from memory is one of the highest-yield review techniques available.

Friday — Day 47 Full-Length Practice Exam 2: Complete a second 180-question timed practice exam. Activity: Score and compare results to Practice Exam 1. Per-domain improvement should be visible. Investigate any domain where performance declined.

Saturday — Day 48 Review Practice Exam 2: Address all incorrect answers. Prioritize conceptual errors over vocabulary errors at this stage. Activity: Final formula sheet review — reproduce all 25 Appendix A formulas from memory. Verify against the appendix.

Sunday — Day 49 Rest. Confirm exam logistics for the final time: testing center address and directions or remote testing platform login; required identification documents; allowed items and prohibited items; start time and expected duration.

.45.8 Week 8: Final Review and Exam

Monday — Day 50 Light Review Only: Spend no more than 2 hours reviewing your personal notes, flashcards, and the high-yield terms in Appendix B. Practice Questions: No more than 20 questions, completed at a relaxed pace with focus on understanding rationale.

Tuesday — Day 51 Light Review: Review Appendix A (statistical formulas) and the Domain Crosswalk. No new material. Activity: Rest in the afternoon. Engage in a physical activity or relaxing hobby.

Wednesday — Day 52 Rest Day: No study activities. Trust your preparation. Spend time on activities that reduce stress and support good sleep.

Thursday — Day 53 Minimal Review: If you feel compelled to review, limit yourself to one pass through your flashcard deck (flagged cards only) and the formula sheet. Stop by early afternoon. Evening: Set out your identification documents, confirm your testing arrangements, and plan your transportation or remote setup.

Friday — Day 54 Exam Day (or final rest day if exam is Saturday): Follow the exam-day guidance in the section below.

.46 Week Before the Exam – Final Strategies for All Candidates

Final Review Priorities

Regardless of which schedule you followed, the week before the exam should shift away from learning new content and toward consolidating and retrieving what you already know. The research on test-taking performance consistently shows that retrieval practice (attempting to recall information from memory) is significantly more effective than re-reading in the days immediately preceding an examination.

In the final week, prioritize these activities in order:

1. Retrieval practice with flashcards — work through all flagged cards daily, retiring those you answer correctly.

2. Formula reproduction from memory — attempt Appendix A formulas daily without reference; check against the appendix only after attempting each one.
3. Review of incorrect practice exam answers — do not redo questions you answered correctly; focus on the items you missed and ensure you understand why the correct answer is correct and why your original answer was wrong.
4. Domain Crosswalk review — scan Appendix B and define high-yield terms aloud or in writing.

Avoid: starting new chapters, attempting to learn new terminology, changing your study approach radically, or running full-length timed exams in the last 48 hours.

Sleep and Physical Preparation

Sleep is the single most impactful factor in exam-day cognitive performance that is within your control during the final week. Prioritize 7–8 hours per night starting no later than five days before the exam. If you experience anxiety-related sleep disruption, reduce the intensity of evening study and avoid screen use in the 60 minutes before bed.

Physical activity during the study period — even a 20-minute walk daily — has documented positive effects on memory consolidation and stress regulation. Do not suspend exercise during the final week in order to study additional hours; the cognitive trade-off is unfavorable.

Exam-Day Logistics

For in-person testing: Arrive at the testing center at least 30 minutes before your scheduled appointment. Bring two forms of identification as specified by the AHIMA CHDA Candidate Guide (typically a government-issued photo ID). Do not bring electronic devices, study materials, or any unauthorized items into the testing room. Eat a balanced meal within two hours of your exam start time.

For remote proctoring: Log into the proctoring platform at least 15 minutes before your appointment window opens. Ensure your workspace is clear of unauthorized materials as specified in the candidate handbook. Test your camera, microphone, and internet connection the day before. Have a backup internet connection available (mobile hotspot) in case of connectivity issues.

During the Exam

Pace yourself at approximately 1.25 minutes per question on the first pass, which allows time for a complete review of flagged items. Do not spend more than 2 minutes on any question during the first pass; mark uncertain questions and move on to preserve time. Answer every question — there is no penalty for guessing, and an unanswered question is certain to receive no credit.

When reviewing flagged questions, trust your analytical reasoning over your initial gut reaction on factual recall questions, but be cautious about changing answers on scenario-based questions unless you have identified a clear error in your original reasoning. Research on exam-taking behavior shows that initial answers on scenario questions are correct more often than changed answers.

After the Exam

Preliminary score results for Pearson VUE-administered examinations are typically available immediately at the end of the test session. AHIMA will send official score reports within the timeframe specified in the candidate handbook. If you do not pass, the candidate handbook specifies the waiting period before retesting and provides a score report by domain to guide your remediation focus.

If you do pass: congratulations. The CHDA credential requires maintenance through AHIMA's continuing education requirements — review the recertification cycle and plan accordingly so that the expertise you have built through this preparation is maintained and deepened throughout your career.

.47 Mnemonics

Memory aids to help you retain key concepts from this guide. Each acronym summarizes a group of related ideas you will be tested on.

.47.1 DICE

D – Data governance frameworks and policies **I** – Integrity and quality assurance processes **C** – Compliance with regulatory requirements **E** – Enterprise-wide data stewardship

On the CHDA exam, data governance questions test your understanding of how organizations structure accountability for data assets. Remember DICE to recall that governance is not just policy-writing but spans integrity, compliance, and stewardship across the entire organization. When a question describes a hospital implementing a data governance committee, connect it to all four elements.

.47.2 VALID

V – Validity of data elements against defined rules **A** – Accuracy of source documentation and coding **L** – Latency and timeliness of data capture **I** – Internal consistency across data systems **D** – Density and completeness of required fields

On the CHDA exam, data quality is tested through its component dimensions rather than as a single concept. Use VALID to enumerate the five dimensions examiners commonly reference when presenting scenarios about data quality audits, dashboard reliability, or EHR data extraction. A question about a report showing contradictory diagnoses across systems is testing internal consistency, the I in VALID.

.47.3 SMART

S – SNOMED CT for clinical terminology and diagnosis mapping **M** – Mapping between code sets for interoperability **A** – Analytics and reporting built on standardized data **R** – RXNORM and LOINC for pharmacy and lab terminology **T** – Terminology governance to maintain code currency

On the CHDA exam, questions about data standards frequently involve knowing which terminology system applies to which clinical domain. SMART reminds you that SNOMED CT anchors clinical concepts, LOINC anchors laboratory observations, and RXNORM anchors medications, while mapping and governance keep those systems interoperable over time. If a question asks which standard supports semantic interoperability between disparate EHR systems, SNOMED CT and the mapping element of SMART point you to the correct answer.

.47.4 WARE

W – Warehousing architecture including star and snowflake schemas **A** – Aggregation of data from operational source systems **R** – Reporting layers including OLAP cubes and dashboards **E** – ETL (Extract, Transform, Load) pipeline design

On the CHDA exam, data warehousing questions test your ability to distinguish between operational databases and analytical repositories. WARE walks you through the full stack: source systems are aggregated via ETL, stored in a warehouse using dimensional schemas, and surfaced through reporting layers. When a question describes slow query performance on a clinical data repository, think of the R and W layers of WARE and whether the schema design or aggregation strategy is the cause.

.47.5 PRISM

P – Predictive modeling using regression and risk stratification **R** – Retrospective analysis of historical claims and outcomes **I** – Inferential statistics including hypothesis testing and p-values **S** – Sensitivity and specificity in diagnostic performance measures **M** – Machine learning model validation and performance metrics

On the CHDA exam, the analytics domain spans descriptive, inferential, and predictive methods. PRISM reminds you that questions may move across all three levels in a single scenario, asking you to interpret a regression coefficient, evaluate a model's sensitivity, or distinguish retrospective from prospective study designs. Pay special attention to the S in PRISM: sensitivity and specificity appear frequently in questions about screening program data and quality measure reporting.

.47.6 CORE

C – Compliance with HIPAA, CMS, and Joint Commission requirements **O** – Outcomes reporting for quality programs such as IQR and VBP **R** – Regulatory submission formats including HL7 and X12 **E** – External benchmarking against national and regional standards

On the CHDA exam, regulatory and reporting questions tie compliance obligations directly to submission formats and performance benchmarking. CORE reminds you that regulatory work is not only about knowing the rules (HIPAA, CMS conditions of participation) but also about producing outputs in the correct format and comparing institutional results to external standards. When a question presents a scenario about a hospital's value-based purchasing score, connect it to the O and E elements of CORE: outcomes reporting measured against external benchmarks.

www.ingramcontent.com/pod-product-compliance
Lightning Source LLC
LaVergne TN
LVHW062028051126
851858LV00005B/112